THE
WORLD
BEST-KEPT
BEAUTY
SECRETS

THE WORLD S BEST–KEPT BEAUTY SECRETS

Hundreds of Insider Tips from the Worlds of Beauty, Diet and Fashion

DIANE IRONS

Vermilion
LONDON

5 7 9 10 8 6

First published in the United States of America in 1997
by Sourcebooks, Illinois

First published in the United Kingdom in 1998 by Vermilion
an imprint of Ebury Press
Random House, 20 Vauxhall Bridge Road, London SW1V 2SA

Random House Australia (Pty) Limited
20 Alfred Street, Milsons Point, Sydney
New South Wales 2061, Australia

Random House New Zealand Limited
18 Poland Road, Glenfield
Auckland 10, New Zealand

Random House South Africa (Pty) Limited
Endulini, 5A Jubilee Road,
Parktown 2193, South Africa

Random House Group Limited Reg. No. 954009

A CIP catalogue record for this book is available from the
British Library

ISBN: 0 09 181617 3

Printed and bound in Great Britain by
Cox & Wyman Ltd, Reading, Berkshire

Although every effort has been made to ensure that the contents
of this book are accurate, it must not be treated as a substitute
for qualified medical advice. Always consult a qualified medical
practitioner. Neither the author nor the publisher can be held
responsible for any loss or claim arising out of the use, or misuse,
of the suggestions made or the failure to take medical advice.

TABLE OF CONTENTS

Dedication

To my mother and father for their love,
guidance and work ethic

Chapter One
ATTITUDE

You Are What You Project!

Welcome to the best-kept secrets of the world's most alluring women. The models, actresses and celebrities I have been privileged to work with have one trait that causes them to stand out in a crowd – the attitude they project to the world. These women that you see on the street, on the movie screen, adorning the pages of your favourite magazines are not the most beautiful women ever created. But don't tell *them* that!

All women can be truly beautiful. The sad fact of life is that there are some potentially lovely women out there who are holding on to some very old myths. I have worked with 'displaced housewives' who decided to throw all their beauty, health and diet routines away because the routines were too self-indulgent or complicated. So what do they do with their extra time? They spend it adorning their homes or families. Hello? What about adorning the inner house? It is not necessary to give up yourself to love someone else; it is only when you truly love and respect yourself that you can give to others freely.

Make the Time

Create precious time for yourself by setting the alarm clock thirty minutes earlier than usual. Begin rituals for yourself that will become as important to you as breathing. If you really don't think that you have enough time during the day, then take it from the minutes wasted on phone calls, shopping or mindless TV surfing.

Keep It Simple

Begin a 'housecleaning' on your body, wardrobe, handbag, cosmetics and anything else that keeps you from feeling good about yourself and your life.

Stand Up Straight

This sounds so ridiculously simple, but it's one of the most evidential traits of those women we so admire. Stand against a wall with head, shoulder blades and heels touching, and buttocks pushed into the wall. Walk away without changing this position. A great posture is a wonderful beginning for your attitude adjustment.

While you're at it, why don't you pick up those droopy bra straps? This will help 'pick up' both those drooping shoulders and those sagging breasts.

Be the Star of Your Own Show

YOU should be what people notice. Your cosmetics and clothes should not compete for attention with each other, or with you. Stay with the basics, but invent your own style. If you like the colour red, then use it as a consistent accent piece in your wardrobe. Do you have a special collection of brooches or bracelets? Show them off; make them your signature. But definitely do not attempt to wear more than two pieces at a time.

Have It Your Way

After years of telling us what to wear and how to wear it, designers have finally accepted that women are not going to be dictated to any more. Finally, after huge rebellions (along with lagging retail sales) in department stores across the country, there is a choice in hem-lines, fabrics and so much more. The result? If you have great legs, feel free to show them off! If you have a lovely waist, accentuate it with a long and elegant ensemble. Play up your good features, and hide away those 'less-than-perfect' areas.

Make an Effort

You owe it to your self-esteem, your family and friends to try! After all, you don't like to look at a messy house or office all day, do you? Don't you really love and admire majestic works of art? A lovely flower arrangement? Become your own canvas, and recreate yourself.

Learn to Trust Your Mirror

Most of us believe only what others tell us, not what we see in the mirror. That's why we desperately seek compliments and depend on other people's feedback. Real 'beauties' rely on their mirror and accept everything they see. When they behold great hair, they enjoy their 'good hair day'. You won't find these women concentrating on the two pounds they gained from last night's dessert.

Don't Be So Modest

While we are encouraged to go out and look our best, we're not supposed to admit that we're trying. Going that 'extra yard' for beauty is perceived as prideful vanity. In addition, some women worry that they may attract the wrong attention. Wallflowers belong only on walls!

Don't Act or Dress Your Age

Every beautiful woman that I have interviewed seemed to possess the same trait: agelessness. If I hadn't been privy to their backgrounds, I would have been hard pressed to put a 'number' on them. You know who these women are: you see them in a magazine or on TV. You know them to be about your age, but they look so much better. Don't necessarily jump to the conclusion that they've had extensive plastic surgery. That is not always the case. How do you begin your own 'timeless' appearance? Pick up a magazine that might be geared to a different age group.

Shop in a different store or department from the one you normally patronize. Find a mentor – someone whose style you've always admired – to help you develop your new look.

**Almost everything we do is based on appearance.
The pursuit of beauty is as old as time.
Cute babies are held longer.
We love flowers for their beauty.**

Start a Journal

The first step to finding your way back to YOU is to start a daily journal. Keep your daily activities and thoughts as a reliable thermometer to your current state of thinking. Use it to keep track of what you're eating, wearing and feeling.

Set Goals

Don't get overwhelmed in the steps to your transformation. Set standards and goals in baby steps. This is especially important if you've somehow lost yourself along the way. It could be as small as 'I will lose five pounds by the end of the month,' or 'I will devote one hour a day just for me'. Sit back, close your eyes and visualize yourself as slimmer, happier or more assertive.

**Beauty begins with self-acceptance.
Look in the mirror, smile and say, 'Hello!'**

13

Find Your Energy Level

Every person possesses an inner clock. Don't rely on the time of day to tell you when to eat, when to rest, etc. Let your body do the talking! It never fails to give you signs that will tell you what it needs.

**Know when to let go!
You're not in charge of the universe.**

No Brainer

Have one or two outfits that you know make you look terrific and require no thought. Keep no more than five cosmetics that you can take out with you and don't have to be colour co-ordinated. Keep one overcoat that will look stylish, you can wear with dignity and hide anything!

Keep Moving!

Don't stay frozen in time. It is such an easy and comfortable place to get stuck. Keep a look that is absolutely your style, but keep re-inventing that look to keep up with the times. You know who the guilty ones are. You've seen that woman who wears that seventies Farrah Fawcett hairdo, when not even Farrah herself has kept that same look. Or better yet, that friend who was MOD in the sixties and refuses to believe that the revolution is over!

I Dare You

Remember that game we used to play as children? Whether it's just getting a manicure or changing your hair colour, just a little something new or different can create a brand new mind set. Oh yes, of course, you can always change it back if you don't like it. But you may love the new you and wonder why you hadn't tried it sooner!

Learn to Forgive

Get back to self-acceptance. Did you break your diet? That just means that you are human. Why is it that it's so much easier to forgive others and not ourselves? Let it go! When you overspend a bit, maybe that's just what you needed at that time to build your spirits. If you find it difficult to forgive others, remember that even the most well-intentioned person can hurt your feelings. Don't dwell on it. Don't let it stay with you, or it will convert itself into a binge, spending spree, or something far more depressing. Throw it away, and get on with your life TODAY!

Self Portrait

Drawings are our subconscious speaking to us.

Take a pencil or crayon and draw a picture of yourself.

Ask yourself what your drawing says about you.

1. Did you take up the whole page?
2. Are you in the corner?
3. Are any of your body parts missing?
4. Are you wearing clothes?
5. What kinds of clothes are you wearing?

6. Are you wearing shoes?

7. Are any of your body parts out of proportion?

8. What would you name your drawing?

Whenever I speak to groups or work with clients, I often use this self-test. It reveals to us what we need to know in order to change our image and self-esteem.

The most evidential self-portrait results were the ones done by teenagers and homemakers re-entering the workplace. They were most likely to draw themselves without body parts, with grotesque bodies, or as being practically invisible, taking up only a small corner of the page.

Meditation Is a Beauty Ritual

I have had the privilege of working with some big names in the modelling and celebrity world. Each of these great stars possessed the unique ability to go into some kind of trance when sitting in front of that mirror. This is a concept that I have found to be a perfectly relaxing and enjoyable way to start the day.

Chapter Two
SKIN

It all begins from within.
Water . . . water . . . everywhere!
On your face and in your body.

Water is the number one beauty treatment favoured by women of every age. You cannot create beauty without beginning with a clean, clear canvas.

Forget the very expensive mineral waters. If you don't drink at least eight to ten glasses a day, you are depriving yourself of the best beauty treatment on Earth.

Japanese women spend twice as much time and money on their skin as any other women in the world.

Cleansing

The first rule of beautiful skin is to stop overcleansing it. This is an unnecessary habit, especially true of women in the United States. Unless you've been up all night digging ditches (you poor dear!), your face is not dirty. Your morning routine should be nothing more than reactivating last night's moisturizer with a splash of warm water or milk. Why milk? Milk is a lactic acid and will allow your face to receive a natural acid treatment.

Please be aware that many of the acids on the market today are synthetic acids which have caused problems with some women. There have been reports of everything from sensitivity rashes to permanent scarring. Be careful of the chemical acids you use, and when you can, substitute nature's acids in your cleansing routine. In addition to milk, consider these natural acids:

1. Pineapple juice
2. Lemon juice
3. Tomatoes
4. Most citrus fruits

Toning

Toning is your second step, and an important one. The purpose of using a toner is to remove residue soap, moisturizer and oil. You can spend a lot for a toner (up to £15 or more at some cosmetic counters), or you can do what many famous models do. Carry around lemons. They are refreshing and more effective than those silly toners that contain only a little lemon but lots of chemicals.

Other inexpensive alternatives:

1. Rose water
2. Witch hazel
3. Or try the following refreshing tea tonic: Mix 2 teaspoons of green or chamomile tea with 1/2 cup water. Saturate a cotton wool ball, and apply all over the face. Allow it to remain on the skin until it evaporates.

Note: There's never any reason to rinse off this or any toner.

Moisturizing

I am happy to pass on one of the most important ways ever to save money. It is not necessary to spend a lot on a moisturizer. Good basic moisturizers can be found in any chemist. Just learn to read the labels, and look for these low-cost ingredients.

Lipids: Listed as ceramides, cerebrosides or sphingo lipids.

Essential fatty acids: Listed as sunflower oil, grapeseed oil and evening primrose oil.

Sunscreen: Now available in many moisturizers as a step-saver.

The Sun Is Your Skin's No.1 Enemy

You should always make sun protection a priority. Use a sunscreen formulated for your skin along with your moisturizer. Many of the signs of ageing – rough skin, wrinkles, age spots, etc. – are really the result of too much sun. Always apply lots of it – not only to your face but also to neck, hands and hairline.

Tip

Don't buy a vitamin E-, A- or C-enhanced moisturizer. Go to your local chemist, and purchase these vitamins in capsule form. Get as much potency as is available. Prick open the capsule and add it to your moisturizer. You'll get all the benefits of the expensive cosmetic creams without the extra chemicals or expense.

Add Water

You'll find most moisturizers more effective when applied to damp skin. It forms a thin film that will trap moisture in the skin. Evening is the most important time to take care of your skin. The sleeping hours are when your face is away from make-up, dirt, pollution, etc., and is free to rejuvenate. Your evening regime is also effective and useful in de-stressing your entire psyche to prepare you for the best treatment of all: beauty sleep.

Just Follow These Steps:

1. Cleanse

Make it easy on yourself, your skin, and your purse by using just one product to remove both makeup and dirt. If your skin is dry, use a lotion or cream-based product that leaves behind emollients (it will feel like a light film on your face). If your skin is 'normal to oily', use a gel cleanser or a very mild facial soap. Even though your skin may be very oily, be sure to use a gentle soap like Neutrogena or Dove. Never use a deodorant soap on your face or neck. If your skin is particularly sensitive, don't even use it on your body!

2. Exfoliate

I cannot overstate the need for this step. What is exfoliating? It is very much like peeling an onion or removing tiles off a roof. Exfoliating is necessary to get blood flowing into the face, as well as to remove grime.

Here's what to use:
Take a teaspoon or two of sugar (unrefined sugar works the best), add a couple of drops of olive oil to create a spreading condition, and gently rub it into the creases of your face.

Open a packet of instant oatmeal, mix it with water and create a paste. Rub this mixture into your face, and rinse off the residue. I would suggest that you use instant oatmeal on your face, and the traditional old-fashioned oatmeal to exfoliate the entire body.

Rub sea salt (available in health food shops) all over both your body and face. You'll love its invigorating effects.

3. Masks

My favourite face mask is the result of my most memorable investigative reporting story. I had been informed that those very expensive spas that charge hundreds of pounds for 'herbal wraps' were using mud. Now the inside 'scoop' is that these 'chichi' places were not using some exotic mud from the Dead Sea, but a formula created from *cat litter*.

Okay, we've all heard of clay masks. Clay is perfect for detoxifying the skin. What I discovered is that these so-called 'mud' or 'clay' treatments used by some salons are nothing more than cat litter. The kind you want is 'fuller's earth', pure and simple; the bag must be marked '100% Natural Clay'. It cannot contain any chemicals, additives or clumping materials. The good news is that this type of cat litter is generally the least expensive on the market.

How to use it:
Take about a tablespoon of the dried clay and reconstitute it with a small amount of water. Mud is mud is mud! I don't care if it comes from the great springs of Italy (and if it does, you'll spend about £40 a pot) or from your local supermarket. At less than £2 a bag, detoxify your entire body with it. I have worked with the most fabulous celebrities who swear by my cat litter facial, including top make-up artists. Although they love this facial, they know that their clients may be a little reticent to try such an unorthodox facial. So they pour the cat litter into an attractive container. You might want to do the same at your house to avoid strange looks. Potpourri jars make delightful hiding places for your new find.

I have demonstrated this several times on American TV shows with people from the audience, and not one person has ever told me that it felt anything but absolutely refreshing. It actually possesses a kind of pleasant, minty feel. Minerals in the mud also benefit the skin.

Please don't try to use the mud from your garden. Real mud is dirty and contains organisms that harbour diseases.

Ultimate Cleansing Mask

Take 170g (6oz) fine oatmeal. Add 3 drops of almond oil, 240ml (8fl oz) of milk and 1 egg white. Continue to blend together. Rinse off after 20 minutes.

Other Face Masks to Try

Mayonnaise

Apply whole-egg mayonnaise on your face (right from the jar) for about 20 minutes. Rinse with cool water.

Peach & Brandy

Mash up a peach (use ripe, tinned or frozen), and mix in a tablespoon of brandy. Leave it on for 20 minutes, and rinse off.

Tomato Mask

For oily skin, mash up a ripe tomato and leave it on for 15 to 20 minutes. Rinse with warm (not hot) water.

Banana Mash

Mash up a very ripe banana Add just enough honey to make a soft pulp. Apply over face and hair. This is such a great firming mask that ageing movie stars have been known to put it in the cups of their bras to make their breasts 'perky'.

23

Just make sure that you don't add too much honey and that you use a sturdy bra. I recently did a TV show, where I attempted to use a lacy bra. Needless to say, it was a little messy!

Honey Mask

Apply pure honey (straight from the pot) to your face and neck. Allow it to set until dry (about 15 minutes). Rinse with very warm water.

Milk of Magnesia

Apply it straight from the bottle. Let it dry for about five to ten minutes. Rinse off with warm water.

Gently pat face dry with fluffy towel.

Pepto Bismol

This is a face mask particularly suited for those with sensitive skin. In the same way that this product coats the stomach, it gently caresses the face. Apply it straight from the bottle with a cotton bud. Allow it to dry and rinse with cool water. It's as refreshing as a cool summer breeze.

Top Secret Tips

To Revitalize and Nourish the Skin

Soak whole French beans or lentils (fresh are best) overnight. Mash and add a small amount of honey. Apply over face and neck. Leave it on for about five minutes and rinse with tepid water.

Tone Up Tired Skin

Make up a smooth pulp of crushed cucumbers, and gently pat all over face and neck. Pull up your hair and apply a little bit behind the ears and behind the neck. This facial is absolutely fabulous for oily skin and clogged pores.

Mix 60ml (2fl oz) vodka with the juice of one fresh lemon. Dab it on the face, neck and chest area with a cotton bud. It's not necessary to rinse off. Let the air evaporate it. The less rubbing that you do to the face, the better.

More Beauty Tricks from the Kitchen Cupboard

Clove Oil Cleanser

Combine equal amounts of clove oil (a natural astringent), chamomile (to maintain skin pigment) and eucalyptus (decongests the skin). Massage gently into the skin by making a circular motion with the tips of your fingers, and rinse.

White vegetable fat

In the States, many beautiful women use this to remove makeup and as a highly effective moisturizer. Hospitals there even use it to treat psoriasis and eczema.

Wheat Germ Oil

Available in health food shops and some supermarkets, wheat germ oil is effective in keeping the skin elastic, and preventing and treating stretch marks. Pregnant women should definitely use it in the tummy and breast areas.

25

Sweet Almond Oil

Available in health food shops, almond oil is ideal for removing makeup, helping eyelashes grow, and as a moisturizer for extremely dry skin. It also soothes sunburned skin.

Bathing

Add some bicarbonate of soda to your bath (about half a box). It will soothe itching skin, irritation and sunburn.

Use Epsom salts (about 230g [8oz]) to relax muscles and relieve swelling.

Try some fine or pinhead oatmeal in the tub to get rid of sunburn.

Apple cider vinegar in the bath will invigorate the body and fight fatigue.

Adding a spoonful of honey to a bath is said to help insomnia.

Combine a cup of instant milk powder with three drops of almond oil. Soak for at least 15 minutes, then using a coarse face cloth or loofah, rub vigorously to exfoliate (remove) dead skin. Your skin will absolutely glow and shine!

Should you start to feel a cold coming on, take a teaspoon of mustard powder and add it to a hot bath. You just might fight off the cold.

Orange slices in the bath are uplifting and beat any aromatherapy available today.

Through the ages red wine has been used as a beauty treatment. Since it is a tannic acid, many beauties use it as an acid-based toner.

Sharing Beauty Treatments with Our Animal Friends

For years models have been sneaking into feed supply stores and equestrian shops for udder cream and hoof conditioner. Now these beneficial products are being sold in chemists and superstores everywhere.

Hoof conditioner is used for horses. However, it softens cuticles, heels and other rough spots. Horse trainers came upon this terrific product by seeing their own positive results. It seems that their nails and cuticles were stronger, longer and more resilient.

Udder cream is an emollient used to soothe those poor cow's udders that take such a licking in those milking machines. This stuff is wonderful on chapped lips and as extra protection during cold weather on hands and face. It's a 'must' for skiers.

One of the oddest moisturizers ever to hit the cosmetic market is Kalaya Oil. It is derived from the 'fat back' of the rare Australian bird, the emu. This moisturizer lessens the sign of ageing by trapping moisture in the skin.

Expert Tip

To get the most from a facial product, rub it between your hands before applying. This action produces heat, making any cosmetic more spreadable.

Moisturizer Know-How

1. Don't over-moisturize. Use cream on specific areas. You may not need it all over your face. The cheeks and forehead tend to be drier than the chin.

2. Choose the right formula for your skin type. More than half of all women mis-diagnose their skin type, believing it to be very oily or very dry. It's highly unusual for a woman's skin to be either. If moisturizer is too heavy, the result is clogged pores. Moisturizing techniques need to be changed as the seasons change.

3. Get more from your moisturizer by circulating the skin. Gently tap the face by pretending your face is a piano, and you're 'playing' it.

4. Any moisturizer can be stretched by first applying a film of natural vegetable oil as a base.

5. Wait until a moisturizer is completely absorbed before applying foundation. However, if a foundation is a bit dry, moisturizer can loosen it up a bit. The foundation will go on more smoothly.

Cellulite

We now know that diet works and thigh creams don't when it comes to cellulite. So what else can we do besides just staring at it? Here are some simple steps:

1. Eat lots of fresh fruit and vegetables (preferably raw).

2. Keep away from processed foods.

3. Drink lots of water to clean cells of toxins.

4. Stay away from fizzy drinks (even low-calorie).

5. Avoid alcohol, which negatively affects the liver, the body's main detoxifier and filter.

6. Try to walk or jog at least three times a week for 30 to 45 minutes.

7. Scrub the skin with a bristle brush or loofah. Brush in slow sweeps, always towards the heart. There are gloves and mitts available to do this, but they're not necessary. Try to do this at least five minutes a day.

   Models are using their morning coffee grounds to massage their cellulite areas. The main ingredient in expensive cellulite creams is caffeine, so this makes lots of sense. Simply sit on the edge of your bathtub, and rub the coffee grounds into those problem areas. It could get messy, so make sure that you have a few newspapers laid out under you!

8. Copy the expensive herbal wraps offered by top spas. Mix a cup of cooking oil with 240 ml (8fl oz) of grapefruit juice and 2 teaspoons dried thyme. Massage into hip, thigh and buttock areas. Cover with clingfilm to lock in body heat. For extra results, lay a heating pad over each area for about five minutes.

Stages of Cellulite

Do you have it? How bad is it? Cellulite does have a way of progressing like a bad fungus.

Test

Cellulite can be diagnosed by using the skin pinch-and-roll technique. Gently take a large fold of normal skin and rub it between your thumb and forefinger. The skin will appear smooth.

Now repeat this test on areas where you think you have cellulite. You may have cellulite in the following stages:

Stage 1

The skin will show no visible signs, but bruises and cuts may be slow to heal in this area.

Stage 2

Looking closely at the skin, you'll see broken veins and skin discolouration. Bruises will appear after a small hit. When pinched, the skin will feel thicker and slightly tender with slight ripples.

Stage 3

Even without pinching the skin, you'll see evidence of an orange peel appearance.

Stage 4

The skin will appear puckered, and is cold to the touch. Broken veins will be present, and bruising can occur spontaneously.

Stage 5

Not only will you feel cold areas, but hot areas will also be evident.

Stage 6

Large lumps of fat are honeycombed in fibres, distorting the appearance of the cellulite area.

Quick Skin Pick-up

Do you need a quick glow to your skin and an all-over healthier look? Bend over at the waist, as far as you can possibly go, and hold to the count of thirty. Scientists have proven that this very simple stance boosts circulation to both face and scalp, speeding up the turnover of skin cells and reducing the possibility of spots. Benefits vary depending on the time of day you choose.

Morning: It helps you to focus on a busy day and awakens the mind and body.

Noon: This is the time for a midday boost.

Night: It helps you unwind, and gets your heart rate and your breathing back to where they should be.

Try to get your head in the proximity of your knees. It's okay to bend your knees until you get used to the position. Steady the stance by clasping your hands behind your back. Still can't seem to do it? Just lie over the side of your bed (head down).

Aids for Blemished Skin

Oatmeal

Yoghurt

Strawberries

Tea tree oil

To Squeeze or Not to Squeeze

If you decide to squeeze a pimple, be very gentle; pressing until it bleeds may rupture tissue and cause scarring. Make sure that skin is clean and warm, wrap your fingers in tissue, and apply light pressure. Dab over it with tea tree oil.

Tip

Retin-A is doing for stretch marks what it has done for the face. Researchers have found that women using this prescription drug for facial problems or stretch marks reduced the stretch marks by 14 per cent after six months of continued use.

Fade Cream

Make your own concoction to lighten age spots and sun-damaged upper chest. Mix the juice of 1 lemon, 1 lime, 2 tablespoons of honey and 60ml (2fl oz) of plain yoghurt. Gently massage into each spot. Use at least once a week.

Face Lift

There are ways to lift your face, on both a cumulative and a temporary basis. For years models, actors and actresses have been relying on the shark's liver oil and yeast contained in hemorrhoidal creams. These are the same ingredients that can be found in expensive 'firming' creams sold at expensive cosmetic counters. What these creams do for those other areas (takes down the swelling and shrinks tissues) is what they also do for undereye bags, droopy jowls, etc. Makeup artists won't do a makeover without it. Rock stars, Hollywood's big names and other celebrities won't go on the road without a supply of it. Many of the people you believe have had plastic surgery have been using it for years.

If you object to the medicinal smell, simply mix it with a small amount of your regular moisturizer. If you need to use it just before going out, dab a little perfume in front of each ear to diffuse any signs. I once interviewed a very handsome actor in his mid-fifties, and could not get over how great he looked. However, I was aware of a certain aroma that I recognized wafting from his direction. If you find that this product works for you, I suggest that you use it at night in the privacy of your own bedroom.

If you are heading out to a special event, and want to tighten your face a bit, use this quick fix:

Beat 1 egg white to a froth. Apply all over face, paying special attention to the eye area, chin and jaw. Allow it to dry (it should take no longer than ten minutes), and ever so lightly rinse it off. Don't waste your money on temporary lifting creams. The egg white lift is just as effective as any 'face lift in a bottle' I have ever tried.

Eyes

Thin cucumber slices used as compresses over closed eyes will relieve soreness and puffiness.

Raw potato slices contain potassium to take away dark circles under the eye.

Inexpensive tea bags (make sure that they're cool to the touch) on the eyes make good eye refreshers because of the tannic acid. Don't use herbal tea bags, because most don't contain tannic acid. Try such brands as Tetley's and PG Tips, or generic brands.

Neck

The neck is often one of the most neglected areas, yet it's the first place where the signs of ageing appear. A certain amount of wrinkling and sagging is inevitable, but there is a lot you can do not only to improve the appearance of your neck now, but to minimize future problems.

Always take your cleanser and creams over the entire throat area, rinsing thoroughly. Make certain to apply all creams with firm upward strokes.

Knees and Elbows

The skin on knees, elbows and heels can easily look discoloured and dead. Here's a bleaching mask that really works wonders. Don't even think of wearing a short skirt without first applying this mixture.

Add the juice of 3 lemons to 90g (3oz) of powdered milk. Use just enough water to make a thick paste. Leave the mixture on for 20 minutes. Scrub off briskly with a loofah or sponge.

Chapter Three
HAIR

A Good Hair Day

So what do you want from your hair? You probably want
it to behave. You want it to have volume. You want it to
shine. That's just how you decide what you need in a hair
product. The number one question I'm asked when it
comes to hair:

**'Is there a difference between expensive hair
salon products and ordinary items?'**

After all these years of research, I still find that there are
no quick answers. I have tried them all (and have the split
ends to prove it), yet have not come up with anything that
beats the natural-based formulas.

Because everyone's hair is unique, it is necessary to experiment a bit. The key is to purchase the smallest size available (travel sizes are ideal), and see what works. We've all
seen the big sales and cut out the coupons. What good is
a big vat of that product going to be if it makes your hair
look like a miniature haystack?

Here's all you'll need for beautiful hair. And I pray that
you never again overspend, buy a useless product or have
a 'bad hair day'.

Find a Stylist You Like and Trust

Ask a friend or acquaintance whose hair you admire.

Pay a little extra to book the salon's master stylist. This is a stylist who has extra training and may also teach or lecture.

If you are done in less than 30 minutes, move on. That's not enough time.

Enter the salon with a specific goal (take a picture along if you need to, but try to be realistic).

Use the Right Shampoo

There are very specific shampoos on the market today to help you make your hair be the best it can be.

Occasionally add a couple of caplets (capsule-shaped tablets) of vitamin E to your inexpensive shampoo for extra nourishment.

There are very good shampoos that perform more than one task.

Use inexpensive brands to strip off extra mousse, gels, etc., at least once a week.

Condition When You Need To

You probably need to deep condition (10 to 30 minutes) only once a week.

Your facial moisturizer can double as a hair conditioner.

If your hair is extremely dry, allow a little conditioner to remain in your hair. The excess will be rubbed off during the towel-drying process.

The Grand Finish

Mousse is a good ending product for fine hair.

Gel is great for control, but should be used in small amounts.

Hair spray should be used at least 25cm (10in) away from the sides of the head, and about 13cm (5in) from the top.

Always use your fingers as a styling aid while using these products.

Back to Nature

Egg Shampoo

Beat 2 eggs in a cup of warm water. Massage the mixture into wet hair. Leave on 5 to 10 minutes. Rinse in tepid water.

Caution: If you rinse in hot water, the eggs could scramble right in your hair and be impossible to get out!

Lather & Strengthen

Mix an egg into your regular shampoo.

To Thicken Hair

Add a tablespoon of powdered gelatin to your shampoo.

Hair Shiners

60ml (2fl oz) lemon juice added to 120ml (4fl oz) water for light hair.

60ml (2fl oz) vinegar added to 120ml (4fl oz) water for brunettes.

Use as a final rinse.

Conditioner for Dry Hair

Mix 1 egg, 1 teaspoon honey and 2 teaspoons olive oil. Apply to wet hair. Cover with a shower cap or layer of clingfilm. Leave on for at least 30 minutes before shampooing out.

Nourishing Hair Pack

Here's what to do with an overripe avocado:

Mash it up and blend through dry hair. Leave the mixture on for 30 minutes. Shampoo thoroughly.

Yoghurt Conditioner

Use plain yoghurt as a conditioner/final rinse.

Rub in after shampooing. Leave on 20 minutes. Rinse with warm water.

Hot Oil Treatment

Mix 240 ml (8fl oz) olive oil and 60g (2oz) butter. Microwave for one minute. Leave on 20 minutes. Shampoo.

Oily Hair Treatment

Add 60ml (2fl oz) aloe vera gel to 120ml (4fl oz) shampoo. Mix well and apply.

Damaged Hair Repair

Mash a ripe banana and mix with a few drops of almond oil. Massage entire head. Leave on 15 minutes. Rinse thoroughly.

Dry Hair Treatment

Mix 1 tablespoon honey to 2 tablespoons shampoo. Shampoo as usual.

Natural Colour Enhancers

Light Hair

Brew a cup of very strong chamomile tea. Let it cool to lukewarm. Spray or comb into dry hair. Leave on about 20 minutes. Shampoo and rinse.

This will give a colour lift to blonde or light brown hair.

Dark Hair

Brew an espresso or other strong coffee. Add to dry hair. Leave on 30 minutes.

This will add sparkling highlights to black or dark brown hair.

Natural Styling

Flat beer is a cheap but effective styling tool. Pour a small amount in a plant mister. Squirt on before setting hair. Don't worry, the smell disappears when your hair dries. Beer will also give life to a tired perm or to naturally curly hair that tends to droop. In these instances, you would spray the beer on dry hair and scrunch the style into shape.

My beautiful colleagues who are also devout environmentalists swear to me that the following works better than any hair spray:

Dissolve a tablespoon of sugar into a glass of hot water. Allow it to cool, and use in a plant mister.

Rules for Highlighting Hair

1. Stick to gold or amber streaks if you have dark blonde or brown hair, and gold or strawberry streaks if you have auburn hair.

2. Don't put highlights too close together.

3. To brighten your complexion, add a few subtle highlights to your fringe and the hair at the sides of the face.

4. To make hair look thicker and fuller, brush highlights along the curves of your cut or on natural curls and waves.

5. To give the illusion of lighter hair, brush highlights throughout your hair, concentrating on your hairline, parting and fringe.

6. Bobs and layered cuts are best suited to highlighting.

7. Condition regularly, but avoid hot-oil treatments. They tend to strip colour.

Dandruff

Vitamin E capsules or vitamin E oil, rubbed into your scalp, will take away those ugly flakes.

Aloe vera gel applied all over your head will work immediately. Let it set for about five minutes, shampoo and rinse.

I interviewed the world-famous hair stylist to the stars – Dusty Fleming of Beverly Hills, who provided me with a unique dandruff shampoo:

Mash 30 aspirin tablets. Add to any bottle of shampoo. No need to refrigerate.

Tip

Any strong dandruff shampoo will work in an emergency to remove extra colour from chemically treated hair. Use it in a pinch when you leave your solution on too long.

Dry Cleaning

When shampooing is not an option, use either 2 tablespoons of cornflour or 1 tablespoon of talcum powder and brush through the hair.

Colouring Tips

1. Women with pink complexions should avoid shades of red or golden blonde. Use ash tones to neutralize your colouring.

2. If your complexion is creamy white, pick dark shades (brown, black or burgundy). They make the skin look luminous.

3. Sallow complexions should stay away from yellow, gold or orange tones. Try deep reds and burgundies instead.

4. Starting at age forty, choose one shade lighter than your natural colour.

5. Dark-skinned women should stay close to their natural hair colour to complement the skin's tone.

Hair Rules to Live By

1. The shorter your forehead, the longer your fringe should be.

2. Protect your hair, as well as your skin, from the sun. Use a sunscreen on hairline partings. Lip balm will also work.

3. To remove residue completely from hair, combine equal amounts of bicarbonate of soda and shampoo. Let set for five minutes.

4. Occasionally shampoo hair with mild washing-up liquid to get rid of product buildup.

5. Don't smile when the hairdresser is cutting your

fringe. Smiling raises your forehead, and your fringe may be cut too short.

6. Don't cross your legs during cutting. It will make you sit unevenly, and one side of your hair may end up longer than the other.

7. Don't try to style soaking wet hair. Get it 80 per cent dry first.

8. For extra lift, hold your head upside down while drying.

9. A volume brush, with a hollow head and widely spaced bristles, will give your hair more volume.

10. Tease your hair with a toothbrush or baby comb. The small bristles will add a lot of volume to small sections of hair.

11. Use a ponytail to create an instant facelift.

12. Reactivate a style by squirting with spring water.

13. Never wash hair with hot water.

14. Always use a hot curling brush to dry hair. The metal locks in heat to make hair dry faster, and tames and polishes hair by smoothing cuticles.

Tip

Take a strand test to make certain that you're using the correct shampoo for your hair type.

Does it snap easily? Your hair is fine or oily.

Is it hard to break? Your hair is coarse or dry.

Wet Hair Woes

Here's a way to leave the house with damp hair and style!

If hair is wet, run styling lotion or gel throughout. Squirt hair spray onto brush, and brush hair back, letting the sides curve down. Finish with more spray.

Never go to bed with wet hair!
No, I'm not kidding!

What do mouthwash, fabric conditioner and wine have to do with hair? They're unconventional hair treatments that REALLY work! Read on!

Red Wine

Neutralize the green colour caused by chlorine by dabbing a little red wine onto the hair. Use it as a precaution before entering the pool. Use it before shampooing.

Mouthwash

Mix 60ml (2fl oz) mouthwash and 240ml (8fl oz) water. Apply to scalp as a cleaner. Use after shampooing.

DO NOT RINSE OUT!

Fabric Conditioner

The best leave-in conditioner is nothing other than laundry room fabric conditioner. It's very strong, so be sure to dilute it.

Suggestion: 230ml (8fl oz) water, 115ml (4fl oz) normal-strength fabric-conditioner.

Experiment with different conditioner scents for your own personal hair 'signature'. Save £££££ over expensive hair products!

Dark-skinned Women

Jojoba oil slicks hair back beautifully!

Conditioning is vital, as hair tends to be dry and brittle.

Copper and chestnut are good colour options for warm or amber tones.

Don't blow-dry hair too often. Let it air-dry whenever possible.

A paddle brush is perfect for keeping hair at its most manageable.

Texture is key to controlling style.

Allow only the most experienced hands to handle weaves.

Dark-skinned women look great in hair colours of deep wine, red or blue-black.

Chapter Four

MAKE-UP

Making Up Is Not Hard to Do!

Everyone has time to make her face more attractive. This is always the key to applying any cosmetic. The purpose of a beauty product should be to make the face look livelier, more interesting, younger, prettier or more polished. Making up your face means looking like YOU, but even better! This chapter has all you need to know to maximize your best assets while minimizing any defects. I'll show you how to do it whether you have 20 minutes or 20 seconds. You DO have time to show your best face to the world.

Always Apply Make-up to a Clean Face

For the best results always start with a fresh face. Think of your face as a blank canvas. You are the artist, and you *must* start with a clean slate. Your make-up will go on more smoothly, more evenly, and will last much longer.

How Much Time Should You Spend on Your Make-up?

15 minutes?
10 minutes?
5 minutes?
2 minutes?

No matter where you're going, your usual routine should be no more than 15 minutes. The trick is to change your routine. There is no way that you can apply 15 minutes of cosmetics into a quick 5-minute regime. You can still look pretty good in just a couple of minutes with my streamlined techniques. There's just no excuse for looking naked, tired or 'war-painted' any more.

The 15–Minute Face

Here's how to apply your make-up when you've got time to create a total look that can take you through the entire day.

Foundation

A good foundation is the hardest-working cosmetic you will ever purchase. Choose one that is right for your skin type. An all-in-one foundation that gives adequate coverage is the combination liquid/powder duo found at every price level. I especially like the lower-cost lines found in Cover Girl, Revlon and L'Oréal. They're less drying than the more expensive brands, and you don't have to wet them to get a flawless finish.

Do you look good in pure white? Look for 'cool' shades.

Do you look better in cream or off white? Choose 'warm' tones.

Take a coral lipstick and a pink lipstick. If your skin more closely resembles the pink, you have pink undertones.

The closer match to the coral means that you have a 'yellow' undertone.

Now you can take this knowledge and confidently choose your own colour at the chemist.

I can't begin to tell you how many complaints I have heard from women who have been given the wrong colour by those so-called 'experts' behind the cosmetic counters. It's time for *you* to become your own expert. After all, who's been looking at that skin in every kind of light imaginable for all these years? Furthermore, if you make a mistake at the chemist, it's easy to go back and get the next shade (lighter/darker) or even to blend the two at a far less exorbitant price.

1. Apply foundation with fingers or a sponge. When you're searching out a look that's more 'natural', your fingers are the best make-up tool. The warmth of your fingers allows your foundation to spread quickly and more evenly. You'll also have more control.

2. Start at the under-eye area. This is where coverage is needed the most.

3. Blend all over the face, including lips. Sweep more heavily over flaws. Go lightly over your 'good' areas to even out the colour.

Eyebrows

The eyebrow is the frame of the face. It is easy to 'lift' the eye with a couple of quick strokes. Many great beauties are known for their distinctive eyebrows (think Brooke Shields, Cindy Crawford and Joan Crawford).

Control your eyebrows with an old toothbrush or an old washed mascara wand.

Which Tweezers?

Thin Tip: Good for grasping small, fine hairs and getting at ingrown hairs.

Slanted Tip: Versatile tweezer affording maximum control.

Square Tip: Best used for removing coarse hairs or several hairs at a time.

Myth: Never pluck above your brow.

Whoever thought of that one? You pluck where you need to pluck!

I once did a make-over on a woman who had these ugly hairs sticking up on her forehead. When I asked her why she didn't pluck them out, she recited to me this silly old outdated 'don't touch those hairs above the eyebrow' rule.

Technique

Brush the brow upwards and outwards to define the natural line. Tweeze under the brow to form an arch. Soften the sting by rubbing the area with an ice cube. If you're completely 'clueless' on what shape to make your eyebrow, cut out an eyebrow from a magazine, and stencil it on top of your own. Tweeze to trace the prototype.

Expert Tip

To get a professional-looking eyebrow, follow these steps.

1. Brush brows down, using a toothbrush or lash comb.

2. Fill in with a soft pencil.

3. Spray a toothbrush with hair spray.

4. Brush brows back up and into place.

Eyes

Step One

Brush medium-toned shadow in a neutral shade over the entire lid. Deepen colour in the crease and slightly above the outer corner of the eye, using a kohl pencil or darker shadow dipped in water. Smudge together to eliminate any unnatural-looking lines.

Step Two

Lightly powder lashes to give mascara a coat to cling to. Line lids as close as possible with a pencil or liquid liner. Brush on the first coat of mascara. Comb through to separate hairs. Powder over liner in a shade just slightly lighter than the liner. Powder under eyes to complete the look.

Secrets of Eyebrows

Eyebrows look best when filled in with a soft

pencil or powder. The modern brow is neither too

thick nor too thin. Undecided? Go to a professional

for your first plucking. It's most effective to work

in a bright, natural light when tweezing. Soften

the look of the brow by patting lightly with powder.

You can use eye shadow to lighten a brow.

Applying False Eyelashes

False eyelashes should be applied after foundation and eyebrows.

1. Powder eyelids.
2. Curl eyelashes to blend in with false ones.
3. Apply adhesive to false lashes, being sure not to touch the lashes themselves.
4. Use a small stick (a toothpick works well) to be more precise.
5. Make sure that the lashes match by starting to fix them at the outer corner.
6. To blend false and natural lashes, apply a deep liquid liner over both.

Secrets

To make the whites of your eyes look brighter, use a light blue pencil under the eyes. Blue eye shadow lightly applied under the eyes works just as well.

Separate clumpy eyelashes with a lash comb, available at chemists.

To get the best curl in your eyelashes, use a blow dryer to heat an eyelash curler for about five seconds before using.

If you need to go from day to evening without starting from scratch, apply an eye foundation before the shadow.

Use waterproof formulations whenever possible.

Always wipe wands off before using to prevent clumping.

When applying mascara to bottom lashes, hold a tissue under the lashes so that mascara doesn't end up on the skin.

Are you an totally cack-handed when it comes to lining your eyes? Use a shadow as liner, or steady your hand by leaning your elbow on a table when applying.

More Secrets . . .

Make your eyeliner last each time you sharpen it by putting it in the freezer for at least 15 minutes prior to sharpening. This will ensure a perfect point with no crumbling.

Bend the tip of your mascara wand until it's angled to resemble a dentist's mirror. The wand will be easier to control, and the brush will give better coverage.

Pull your eyelid taut when applying eyeliner.

It actually helps to keep your mouth open when applying eye make-up. It keeps you from blinking.

Always apply liner in short, feathery strokes.

Neutral shadows are the most flattering to the eye.

Create a V-shape with a soft powder at the outer corner of the eyes to lift.

Applications

Wide-set eyes: To make your eyes look closer together, apply deep-toned shadow to the inner halves of the lids. Light-toned shadow goes on the outer halves.

Close-set eyes: Open up eyes by brushing deep-toned shadow on the outer half of the lids. Blend from the centre of the eyes out and up to just above the crease. Use a light shadow on the inner halves of the lids and just under the brow bone.

Safety Tips

Keep container lids and caps tightly closed.

Keep all applicators clean.

Store eye make-up at room temperature.

Don't let cosmetics sit on top of the radiator.

Use disposable products whenever possible.

Replace products often.

If a product produces an odour, discard it immediately.

Never rest an applicator on a public washbasin.

Never share your make-up.

Lips

Lipsticks have three basic components.

Pigment: Determines the colour.

Emollients: Carry the pigment to the lips.

Waxes: Give the lipstick its shape.
    Choose the best formula!

Matt: The most lasting formulation.
    Not shiny. Flat coverage.
    Caution: Pick one that's not too drying.

Creamy: Looks the best when first applied.
    Gives the most even coverage.
    Available in the widest array of colours.

Stain: Usually contains moisturizing ingredients.
    Gives only a hint of colour.
    Wears off most naturally and discreetly.
    Most likely to have added sunscreen.

Secrets

Use a neutral lip pencil rather than one that matches your lipstick.

Apply lip pencil in dots around the lip, then play 'connect the dots', following the natural lip line.

For a softer lip colour, blend moisturizer into the lipstick.

To change the colour of any lipstick, apply yellow eyeshadow on the lips as a primer. This will warm up any colour.

Blend lip liner and lipstick together on the back of the hand for a longer-lasting look.

If your lipstick tends to 'bleed', apply lipstick first, then line over it to set.

Create your own lip colours by mixing and matching.

Right from the Experts!

To achieve a pouty, sexy mouth, emphasize your top lip by dabbing just a touch of gloss in the centre.

To keep lipstick on while dining, keep lips off utensils. Use your lower teeth and tongue to do the work.

If you feel that your lips are unbalanced, use a lighter coloured lipstick on the smaller lip.

Applying lipstick with a brush will make the tube last longer.

A little bit of red or orange in the centre of the lips makes them look fuller.

After applying lipstick, pucker lips into an extreme 'O'. Cover your finger in a tissue, and poke it into your mouth. Twist away any excess colour that will eventually land up on your teeth.

Bronzing Powder

Ask any beauty what product she would most like to have on a desert island, and the answer would most likely be her BRONZING POWDER. This is the most versatile cosmetic you will ever own. Bronzing is the way to finish your face. Forget blush! I have never seen more beauty blunders than I have with the misuse of blush. I can't begin to tell you how many stripes and circles I have had to wipe off. Use blush improperly and you end up looking like a circus clown or a road marker. This is why I suggest (no, implore) you use bronzing powder to add colour to your face. It's the perfect tool for nonprofessionals to use to contour their faces. Use it on the cheeks, down the sides of the nose (to slim), under the jaw line (to take away a double chin or drooping jowls), and to add colour to the face. You'll find bronzing powder readily available at chemists, cosmetic counters, wherever your budget takes you. But please get some and use it! Why go out in the sun when you can get a better sun-kissed look with this wonderful product? Can you tell it's my all-time favourite cosmetic?

The Five-Minute Face

To look completely set to go in five minutes or less, concentrate on the basics.

Apply foundation as a concealer on shadows and ruddiness.

Apply liner/shadow over and under lids.

Use a neutral lipstick on the apples of cheeks and lips.

The Two-Minute Face

Apply tinted moisturizer all over your face.

Apply a quick coat of mascara.

Apply bronzing gel on eyes, cheeks and lips.

Don't You Dare!

When you're in a rush, don't even try the following:

Liquid eyeliner: Needs time and a steady hand.

False eyelashes: Takes precision, strips, glue and toothpicks.

Plucking: Takes time for the redness to disappear.

Lip liner: You could end up very uneven.

Foundation: Aim for a healthy glow instead.

Expert Tip

Bronzer is absolutely elegant for creating a monochromatic look. Use it to shadow eyes, as a finishing powder for lips, to soften eyebrows and as a finishing powder to set make-up.

Darker Skin Tones

Deeper complexions provide the perfect canvas for creating dramatic looks, but all products need to be carefully chosen and correctly applied to enhance the skin's unique tone and texture.

Foundation

There are more than forty shades between the lightest and deepest of dark skin, so finding the right foundation can be a real challenge. Always test foundation on your cheek or nose. The skin around the outside of the face is often darker than the skin in the centre. Black skin has a lot of yellow pigment, so look for foundations with yellow undertones. Choose oil-free formulations, as darker skin reflects more light and is often slightly oily. Finish with a powder that's either transparent or slightly lighter than your skin.

Eyes

The general rule is that the darker the skin, the deeper the eye colour. This is because darker skin tends to absorb colour. Use rich eye colours like gold, deep grey, purples, russet, copper and brown. Pale pink and beige are enhancing highlighters. If your eyebrows are a little sparse, use dark brown or black pencil to fill them in. Use a kohl pencil to rim your eyes, and a couple of coats of mascara.

Lips

The same rule of 'the darker the skin, the darker the colour' applies to the lips. Red lips are perfect for evening, but choose reds with warm, brown tones, rather than blue undertones, which tend to be too cold. Women with darker skin usually have darker pigmentation outlining their lips, so they have their own natural lip line. If you do find that you require a lip liner, stay in the brown tones.

Blush

Peach or brown tones are most flattering to dark skin. You'll find that pink shades have too much of a blue undertone. For day, use a large soft brush to spread the colour. For evening glamour, use a brown shade a couple of tones darker than your natural skin colour.

Double Duty Cosmetics

Lipstick makes a great cream blush. You'll find it's a perfect way to colour-co-ordinate your face.

A nude pencil is just right to outline lips, cover blemishes and line brows.

Eye shadow doubles as a lip powder.

Mascara can be used to create a beauty mark.

Dark brown eyeliner can be used as a lip pencil.

Dry blusher can be used to seal lips or to change lip colour.

Translucent powder can be used to lighten brows and to seal lipstick.

Concealer hides redness and thins a too-prominent nose.

Powder puffs sprayed with hair spray help powder stay put.

When retouching make-up in the middle of the day, go lightly. Oil from the skin will absorb the make-up's colour and intensify it, making it look artificial.

Pressed powder has a finer texture than loose powder, and looks less 'floury'.

Brush powder only on the centre of the face. The sides of the face are always drier and don't require it.

Chapter Five

MODELS' SECRETS

A Model's Bag

A model's bag is filled with things you've never dreamed of! Here's a sampling of what you would find if you were to peek into the everyday bag of a working model.

P.S.: Every model gets a workout just from lugging the thing around!

Baby Wipes

This is a great tool for both cleansing the face and removing make-up. Baby wipes are hygienic (use them once, and throw them away) and gentle to the face. You'll find that most versions contain lanolin, which is a skin softener. Purchase the convenient travel pack to freshen up at a moment's notice. It's also useful for taking up a stain or deodorant mark.

Hemorrhoid Cream

As mentioned in Chapter Two, it is *the* secret backstage of top runways. We use it on our puffy eyes, along the jaw line and on puffy cheeks. It is an instant face lift, and a favourite of the die-hard party-goers.

Garlic & Papaya Tablets

This is an absolute must when it's necessary to get weight off in a hurry. Garlic and papaya tablets act together as a diuretic and can get up to 2.5kg (6lb) off in a couple of days. Ask your pharmacist for the strongest strength available over the counter. Take two garlic tablets with two papaya tablets before breakfast, lunch and dinner. Eat lightly on these days, staying away from salt. There are 'star' caplets out there on the market with similar ingredients priced at £60 and up. You can buy garlic and papaya tablets in your local chemist or health food shop. Prices vary considerably; but you should be able to get 50 papaya tablets for under £4 and the same number of garlic tablets for less than £5. Of course, being natural supplements, they're much safer than the chemical weight-loss products so widely sold.

Chalk

Here's a natural way to hide stains. Carry white chalk for white clothing, and coloured chalk for all the different colours of your wardrobe. I prefer that you use these natural treatments over chemical stain removers because they are safer for the planet and because many fabrics can be ruined by chemical versions.

White Eyeliner

Models find white eyeliner essential to create a wide-eyed look. Use it along the lash line and softly smudge it with a sponge applicator.

White Eye Shadow

Models use it to create a shimmering face base by mixing it with their foundation. Stroked just under the brow, it lifts the eye.

Vaseline

You can create your own tinted gloss, and save lots of money at the same time. Simply mix any of your favourite lipsticks with a dab of Vaseline.

Eye Redness Reliever

Have I got a way for you to remove spots quickly! In the same way that eye redness relievers take the redness out of the eye, so does it remove redness from pimples. Squeeze out a little on a cotton bud. Hold it on the pimple for ten to fifteen seconds, or until it disappears. Models (and the people who hire them) consider it a tragedy to get a pimple, but it's also important for you when you have that big party, to obliterate those little suckers. This *will* do it, and quickly.

Tights

What do you think models do with ripped tights? They make their very own scrunchies. You know, those fabulous hair accessories that pull your hair back with so much style, but cost a fortune? Here's what you do. Take the tights' leg (the more opaque styles provide more elasticity), and cut at 5–10cm (2–4in) intervals. You'll find that these scrunchies will hold the hair beautifully without any of the stress or split ends that elastic bands can cause.

Erasers

What do models do when they lose an earring back? What do they do when their earring is just too heavy to sit properly on the ear? We take the eraser off a pencil and use it to hold that earring in place. Use this when you drop the back of an earring in your office, etc.

If you should find yourself in a restaurant, simply take a small piece of cork from your wine bottle. It works just as well.

Hair Spray

Hair spray is helpful for keeping your hairstyle in place, but it also keeps tights from running. Spray (lightly, please) a thin film up and down your tights before each wearing.

To keep your make-up in place, close your eyes and, holding the can at arm's length, spray a light mist of hair spray on your face.

BE VERY CAREFUL IF YOU HAVE SENSITIVE SKIN!

Satin Pillowcase

A satin pillowcase is necessary to keep that hair style under control while travelling. Not only will it be an essential when you travel, but you'll enjoy using it at home. Sleeping on a satin pillowcase will help prevent wrinkles while you sleep.

Lemon Juice

Forget the expensive toners. Models carry lemons in their bags to remove residue from their face and to refresh.

Sometimes we carry fresh lemons, but there's only so much one can stuff into those bags. If you do choose to purchase reconstituted lemon juice, make sure that it contains *real* lemon.

Iced Water

You've heard that models drink lots of water. Well that's very true, but only half the story. To get optimum benefits from water, models drink iced water. With iced water, the body needs to use more than 100 calories just to warm itself to room temperature to absorb the water. You are actually using more calories than you are taking in.

Teething Rings

Placed on the eyes, teething rings will reduce any puffiness, and provide a well-rested, wide-awake appearance. Frozen teething rings are a soother for sunburned skin.

Spoons

Here's yet another way to wake up those eyes. Run a spoon under cold water. Hold the spoon over the eye for about thirty seconds. The coolness of the metal 'wakes up' the eyes.

Parsley

Parsley is rich in chlorophyll. It is a major ingredient in leading breath fresheners, such as Clorets. Breath sweetening is more effective when it's done from inside the body. There is a lot of advertising going on now to get people to invest in internal breath fresheners. Again, don't spend a lot for these products. Do what knowledge-able models do to ensure 'kissable' breath. Eat the parsley on your plate at mealtimes, or carry dried parsley in your bag to instantly freshen your breath. Parsley will keep your breath fresher a lot longer than topical fresheners will.

Tea

Tea keeps cavities away! Both green and black tea contain fluoride and polyphenols to prevent plaque from adhering to the tooth's surface. Models drink tea for this very reason, and carry their tea bags faithfully. After models are done drinking their tea, they use their cool tea bags to refresh their eyes. Simply squeeze the tea bag so that it isn't dripping, and gently dab the bags under the eye area. If your face is clean, run over the entire face for a quick pick-me-up!

Unfiltered Apple Cider Vinegar

What a versatile product! It's a great blood purifier when you put a tablespoon in a cup of hot water and drink it. You can use it as an astringent for both your face and your hair.

Toothbrush

Here's an old model's trick that everyone can copy. Brush your lips! Not only does it take away any chapping, but it plumps up the lip temporarily for that sought-after 'pouty' look. A toothbrush is a super jewellery cleaner, getting into nooks and crannies.

Tape

Models always carry double-sided tape to tack up fallen hems, make quick repairs in badly fitting clothing, and 'quick tack' an accessory.

Candles

Carry around small birthday candles. Use them to get a stuck zipper going again.

Colon Cleanser

No, I don't need to elaborate, but there is something to be said for the theory that beauty starts from the inside. Top actresses and great beauties throughout history have used this unconventional beauty/health regime. The legendary actress Mae West was famous for her daily enemas. Her skin was like silk until her death. These cleansers are now extremely popular, and readily available at health food shops in kits and capsules.

Jelly Beans

A jelly bean is a quick energy boost and surprisingly low in calories and fat. Most of these little treats – which are just starting to be carried in British sweet shops and newsagents – contain only 5 or 6 calories each. Compared to a stick of gum (up to 20 calories), it's a pretty good way to snack.

Kelp

Models carry kelp tablets to speed up their metabolism.

Olive Oil

Here is an all-natural substance that models rely on when they're in the sun. Not only does it protect hair from the sun's harsh rays but it is enhanced as super conditioner by the sun's natural heat.

Feverfew

Some super beauties eat feverfew sandwiches to relieve PMS and headaches. I would suggest that you get the tablets.

Rosemary Oil

Rubbed into the temple, rosemary oil relieves pain by relaxing constricted muscles.

Crystallized Ginger

When travelling, models rely on crystallized ginger to prevent motion sickness.

Dandelion Tea

This is used as a diuretic. You can find this product in natural food shops and some chemists. Stay near a lavatory!

Brewer's Yeast

When a spot appears, it can sometimes mean the loss of an important job for a model. That's why models always keep brewer's yeast close at hand. Mixed with plain yoghurt and applied to skin, it can prevent a pimple from coming through.

Surgical Tape

Use surgical tape (available at most chemists) to smooth skin while you sleep. Tape an 'X' between eyebrows, just above the nose. We often make many expressions while we sleep that can cause wrinkling and furrowing.

Lemon Peel

Lemon peel is a great natural mouthwash which is more effective than commercial brands. Combine the lemon peel with a small amount of witch hazel and rinse away.

How Models Get Great Skin

The following tips are from models who must remain anonymous because of contractual agreements.

'I drink a ton of spring water. I don't smoke, and I rarely drink. When I do drink wine, I always choose a spritzer. Before a shoot, I avoid fatty foods and chocolate.'

'I boil some full-fat milk, then let it cool down. I lift off the film that forms on the surface, and apply it to my skin. After it dries, I scrub it off and exfoliate my skin.'

'I drink a power punch every morning. I mix up an equal amount of ginseng, vitamin B-12, wheat grass and royal jelly. Not only is it great for my skin, but it gives me instant energy and helps me last through a whole day of shooting.'

You can find a variety of energizing drinks, both carbonated and still, at health food shops and some chemists.

*'I wash my face with 2 teaspoons of sea salt,
1 tablespoon sesame oil and 1/2 teaspoon
lemon juice.'*

*'I mash up a melon and leave it on my face for about
15 minutes. The melon is rich in beta carotene to combat
cell damage.'*

*'I add a tablespoon of honey to my bath. It invigorates my skin
and leaves it feeling silky.'*

How Do Models Stay in Shape?

*'I eat twice a day. So after toast and coffee in the morning,
I choose between lunch or dinner, depending on my schedule.
I do 500 sit-ups a day, followed by a 5-mile cycle ride or a
40-minute run.'*

– Elle Macpherson

*'I eat a breakfast of fruit, tea and orange juice. For lunch it's
usually diced chicken breast, boiled egg and green salad. My
afternoon snack is tomato juice, black grapes and herbal tea.
Dinner is simply salad and steamed vegetables.'*

– Claudia Schiffer

*'My breakfast is cereal with banana and skimmed milk.
Pasta or salad is usually lunch; sushi, brown rice and
vegetables for dinner. Dairy products go right on my rear
end, so I avoid them.'*

– Cindy Crawford

Source: *Top Model*

Secrets of Taking a Great Picture

Strike a Pose!

Years of taking pictures have yielded a list of do's and don'ts. Whether it's for a business picture, yearbook or that special family event, make your next picture session an absolute success!

What to Wear

Choose plain colours, avoiding patterns, which grab too much attention away from the face.

Wear black and white, with heavier emphasis on black for blondes and white for brunettes.

Avoid jewellery that would distract from the face or that would possibly date the photo.

Avoid clothing that would indicate a season or trend. Stay with classic clothing.

Make-up

Don't use moisturizer under your foundation. It can look extremely 'greasy' in a photo.

Use lots of powder, but make certain it's a matt powder.

If you'll be snapped by flash photography, go heavier on make-up. Flash photography bleaches out cosmetics.

Line lips, and then dip a cotton bud in powder, and run along the line. This will create a mouth that 'pops' out.

Never wear frosted or unusual colours.

Avoid overstyling or 'big' hair. It looks overdone.

Models prefer running to any other exercise. They choose it not only for their figures but for healthy complexions.

Most models agree that on-the-job training is the only way to learn. Most of the most successful models never attended 'modelling schools'.

Chapter Six

HANDS AND FEET

A Secret to None!

Now why would I devote an entire chapter to hands and feet? For many reasons. The first being that I have been witness to the sabotage of a perfect look by the unkempt appearance of raggedy nails, uneven cuticles and 'never thought about it' feet (in sandals no less).

For those who have the time, it is really easy and fun to do your own manicure and pedicure. There are definite tricks to learn that will make you *want* to go the extra step.

I have spoken with employers who have admitted that they have turned down an otherwise qualified job candidate because of a sloppy appearance. That applies to both women and men. With this in mind, take a few minutes, read this chapter, and learn the secrets.

The 8–Step Perfect Manicure

1. File

Using an emery board, file nails straight up at the sides. Don't file sides of nails inward. The thinner your nail, the finer the emery board should be.

2. Cuticles

Apply cuticle softener to the edges of the nail. Massage gently with fingertips. Udder cream (for cows) is an inexpensive cuticle treatment that works well.

3. Soak

Soak fingers in warm, soapy water. If fingers are discoloured or dirty, take a tablet of denture cleanser, and dissolve it in the water.

4. Trim

Using a cuticle pusher/cutter (available at chemists), push the cuticle back, and cut any excess hangnails. Don't cut 'in' to your cuticle, because it will cause it to bleed.

5. Massage

Apply a moisturizer all over the hands, rubbing into the nails and cuticles.

6. Wipe

Dip a cotton wool ball in an astringent (like witch hazel or lemon juice), and remove any excess oil. This is necessary to allow varnish to go on smoothly without bubbling.

7. Base Coat

Apply a base coat or primer, and allow to dry.

8. Final Coat

Brush on a one-coat varnish. Look for the kind that contains both a colour and top coat. It's just as good and a great time saver.

Special Problems

Brittle Nails

Sun damage can cause brittle nails. Always apply sun-screen protection.

Once a week, apply an oil or cream, and wear gloves on your hands overnight.

Choosing a Nail File

One of the ways that you can ruin your nails is by using the wrong nail file. There are files designed for artificial nails, files for buffing and even files for both one-way and two-way filing. Here are some choices:

Emery Board

This is the old stand-by. It's inexpensive and useful for natural nails.

Metal File

It's a practical file that can be washed and re-used. It will leave edges very smooth.

Cushioned File

A practical file because of its dual purpose. The slightly abrasive side shapes natural nails. The smooth surface buffs and finishes them.

The Do-It-Yourself Pedicure

Supplies:

Shower gel for soaking

Varnish remover

Varnish

Wooden orange stick

Foot file

Plastic bags or heavy socks

Tissue

Steps

1. Soak feet to soften.
2. Separate toes with tissue.
3. Apply remover to eliminate oils.
4. File to a square shape. Run the file vertically over the nail to prevent future snags.
5. Apply a base coat (yes, this step is necessary even on a pedicure).
6. Apply varnish.
7. Brush nails with oil to prevent ridges from forming.
8. Allow varnish to dry for 30 minutes.

Problems/Solutions

Thickened Nail Varnish

After you've had nail polish for a while, it tends to thicken. Rather than toss it, turn the bottle upside down, and roll it between your hands. Don't ever add nail varnish remover to thin nail varnish. Although it appears to thin it out temporarily, it will eventually dry the varnish out and spoil whatever is left. When varnish gets so gloppy that the colours separate, it's too old to keep. Get rid of it.

Chapped Hands

Dry, chapped hands are a real problem to anyone who enjoys the outdoors or does heavy housework. One solution is to use udder cream. Neutrogena Norwegian Formula Hand Cream is another effective product; a tiny bit of it goes a long way. Many perfectly polished beauties swear by Vaseline to combat dry skin on hands.

Chipped Varnish

Use a file and smooth out the chipped polish until the ridge is even with the nail. Apply polish only to the chipped area, and allow it to dry. Re-coat the entire nail.

Split Nail

Apply quick-drying glue to the split, and let dry. Smooth with a file or buffer. Mend with a tea bag by cutting a tiny piece from the tea bag. Cover the split, and dot on nail glue. Let dry and smooth with a buffer.

Smudges

Apply varnish remover to smudged varnish to smooth out. Let it dry, and follow up with a thin coat of varnish.

Sounds Fishy

When you're looking for a superior nail enamel, locate the type that contains ground herring scales. This strange ingredient is known in the industry as natural pearl. It gives varnish an extra shine and causes it to stay pure for a longer period of time.

Yellowed Nails

To prevent the discolouration that occurs with nail varnish stains, always use a base coat of superior quality.

Pale Nails

Although pale nails can be hereditary, more often they are the result of poor circulation or anaemia. Take an iron supplement or add iron-rich foods to your diet.

Peeling Nails

Avoid quick-dry varnishes that contain acetone, which can dry out your nails. Always file nails lightly, just enough to shape and keep the layers even. Uneven nails have a tendency to peel.

Brittle Nails

Moisturize with an oil or emollient. There are several on the market, but a vitamin E capsule works just as well.

Dull Nails

After a day or two, varnished nails tend to look a bit dull. Hoof lacquer, the secret weapon of manicurists, keeps nails looking like new. Purchase this product in your local equestrian shop.

Artificial Nails

Although artificial nails can make your hands look more attractive, they can seriously damage your own nails. The worst offenders are the stick-on variety, which cause some of the nail surface to get torn away when they are removed. Another problem is the glue, which can cause an allergic reaction.

Foot Calluses

Always use a pumice stone. Razors and other cutters are not advisable and are not used by most professional pedicurists.

Cracked Hands

Better than lotion, mashed potatoes will solve this frequent problem. Boil a small peeled potato until soft. Mash with 1 tablespoon olive oil. Apply to hands and leave on for 15 minutes. Rinse with cool water.

Aching Feet

Practise picking up small objects like marbles or tiny balls with your toes. Curl toes under, and hold that position for a few seconds. Repeat several times. Alternate walking on the balls of your feet (like a ballerina) and heels every day.

Insider Tips

Let fingers rest at least a day between removing old varnish and applying new. This allows the nail a chance to 'breathe'.

Add $1/2$ teaspoon of sugar to a dollop of hand cream, and massage the entire hand. This smooths and softens.

Always wash hands thoroughly before a manicure. If it's necessary to clean hands after nails are done, use a cleansing pad. Soap and water wash away protective creams left over from the manicure.

Use an old eyeliner brush dipped in nail varnish remover to clean up a messy manicure.

Look for Teflon, the trademarked name that revolutionized the cooking industry, in nail products.

Use a face mask to treat your hands and feet. Hydrating masks work especially well. Gently file nails every other day to keep tips smooth and prevent snags and breaking.

Chapter Seven
FASHION AND STYLE

What Is Fashion?

Here's what you need to know. Style is not fashion, and fashion is not style. You can wear every fashion trend that's come around the fashion bend in the last century and never be stylish. Conversely, you can scoff as fashions come and go and still be the doyenne of style and good taste. Fashion changes by the minute, and we cannot take it seriously. Doing so is a sure sign of becoming a fashion victim. The majority of stylish women I have come across treat fashion with some degree of irreverence. You should too. Trust me, fashion is *not* and never has been brain surgery.

What Is Style? It's Not Being Afraid to Stand Out!

Women of style are not afraid to take fashion risks. They are the ones who will take an article of clothing and wear it in a way it was never intended to be worn. For instance, it's the woman who will wear a classic trousertsuit (maybe it's Armani) and accompany it with a campy T-shirt from her latest holiday.

Style Is Having a Trademark and Being Recognized for It

It could be something as simple as not being seen without that great black jacket. Or maybe it's those brown suede trousers that look chic and appropriate dressed up or down. Sue is a friend who seems to love the combination of navy and pink. She wears it with panache, whether she's going to her son's baseball game (picture old blue jeans and a pink sweater, topped by a classic navy blazer) or a symphony concert (she stole the show by making her appearance in a lovely navy taffeta full skirt, topped by a beautiful frilled pink blouse).

Style Is Not Obeying Silly Fashion Rules

Okay, maybe you just love faux animal prints. You coveted them long before they hit the fashion runways. You have dug through many charity shop bins to add to your collection. Wearing them makes you feel different, etc. Style is having the good sense not to wear more than one piece at a time. Style is knowing not to wear these special pieces to that job interview or to a funeral. Get my point? That is style.

Style Is Knowing When to Stop

Let's take that love for animal prints. The difference between stylish and tacky is wearing one, maybe two pieces, at a time. The secret to being well dressed is underdressing. This allows you to wear distinctive clothing that stands by itself.

Style Is Good Fit

Having a good eye for how clothes fall is crucial to stylish dressing. You should know where those trousers should fall or how that jacket should hang. For example, Adrienne is a beautiful woman who spends an absolute fortune on top designer names. What keeps her from becoming the woman of style she is desperate to be is that she insists on wearing a certain size, no matter how it fits her. Somehow, she has it in her mind that she is a size eight. Yes, she may be a size eight in some designers, but not others. As any stylish woman will tell you, a Calvin Klein size ten just may be a Louis Férand's size six. Try it on!

Style Is Going with What Works for You

If it feels comfortable, like YOU, then you're going to get a lot more wear out of it. This is a fundamental concept of style that you should live with every single day. Even though it's right off the runway, unless you feel confident in it, leave it alone.

The Classics

There is a backbone to fashion known as 'classic dressing'. It is what allows a woman to remain stylish throughout the seasons of her life. These women are not wearing the outrageous fashions seen on the runway. You won't see these women following the fashion editorials in this month's magazines. The looks you see in these arenas are important in that they stimulate our interest in fashion and style. They give us ideas, and they're meant to be talked about, in much the same way as we discuss art. But even the fashion magazines themselves don't mean for every page to be taken literally.

A Classic Wardrobe

Here is my list of classic 'must haves'. These are the things that you can keep twenty or thirty years, with only occasional updates for breakage, change of size or just boredom.

The sheath dress
Gold hoop earrings
Black skirt
Tank top
Well-cut jacket
Basic trousers
Loafers
White cotton shirt
Tank watch
Pearls
Black or white T-shirt
Cardigan

Fashion Don'ts

Here is the ultimate list of a 'never stylish' fashion victim.
I don't care who wears them, how great a buy or how great
it makes you feel. Stay away!

Lace stockings

Sequins during daylight hours

Fishnet stockings or clothing

More than two theme pieces (western, menswear, etc.)

Sleeping bag coats or jackets

Bell bottoms

Baby doll dresses

A skirt shorter than 53cm (21in)

Huge shoulder pads

Sweat shirts

Tracksuits when you're not jogging

Dirty plimsolls

Cheap fabrics

Shoe heels higher than 8cm (3in)

More than two bracelets

More than two earrings in each ear

Transparent clothing

Underwear as outerwear

Ankle bracelets

Acid-washed clothing

Peter Pan collars

Sunglasses indoors

Bra tops

Belly buttons off the beach

Clogs with skirts

Tie-dye

Madras

Camouflage Dressing

No matter what size, age, height or weight you are, you can look younger, thinner and better than ever with the techniques I use when I'm doing make-overs and transformations. When I'm asked to do a TV make-over, invariably the producers ask me not to have the 'transformee' appear 5 kilos (11 pounds) thinner, but hey, let's go for 10 kilos (22 pounds) thinner. When TV ratings are at stake, I have my work cut out for me, and I'd better deliver. Here are my tried-and-true secrets for camouflage dressing which I know will work for you.

After utilizing these tips, you will be assured by your *own* transformation that not all those gorgeous creatures you see in magazines, TV and movies are anorexic, attached to their treadmills, or creatures from another planet. They are just real people who *know* how to accentuate the positive and play down the negative.

Dressing Thinner

1. Match your tights or stockings to your shoes. Legs look longer and thinner when they are toned with skirts and shoes.

2. Pleated trousers conceal tummy bulges, so if this is your problem, stick to those pleats.

3. An A-line skirt emphasizes body length while hiding thighs.

4. Use a shirt like a jacket or a tunic. Choose a generously cut shirt in a heavy or lined fabric. It's an elegant look over slim trousers, flowing gently over every possible sin.

5. Dress in one colour. Wearing one colour from shoulder to shoe streamlines the body. It's called *monochromatic dressing*. If you don't want to limit yourself to just one colour, choose colours that are closely matched. If you really want to look thin, stick to darker colours.

6. If you have a chubby neck, choose v-necklines. They create the illusion of a longer, leaner body.

7. To bring attention to the face and away from the body, wear a choker and matching earrings.

8. A long jacket is a 'pounds parer'. It can make any outfit look elegant while hiding figure flaws.

9. Choose a low-heeled shoe that is cut low on the instep. Stick to a thinner, more graceful heel.

10. A loosely fitted waistcoat can hide a thick waist.

11. Wear belts in a low-slung manner or gently held around the waist.

12. Always wear control top tights with Lycra.

13. A 'body' can eliminate bulge. It also gets rid of unsightly panty lines and fabric pulling.

14. Choose a well-fitted jacket. A look that is too loose or boxy tends to add weight.

15. Simple styling is most slimming. Cuffs, pockets and buttons can add width to the body.

16. Wear prints only at the slimmest part of your body. Stay with smaller rather than big flowery prints.

17. Look for fabrics that drape the body. This would include light wool, cotton and rayon.

How to Spot a Fashion Victim

1. They buy clothes that they have no intention of wearing.

2. They purchase things without first trying them on.

3. They buy more than one of the same outfit in the same colour.

4. They find things in the back of their cupboard, with the tickets still attached.

5. They purchase an item that has nothing to do with their lifestyle, just because it's the latest rage.

Good Jeans

Many women feel that finding the perfect pair of jeans is like searching for the perfect man. There really is something to be said for a great pair of jeans. Some women use them like a scale. They feel that they're in shape when they can fit into their jeans.

Here's What to Like About Jeans

1. Jeans are classless.
   No one can tell how much money you have by your jeans.

2. Jeans are sexy.
   If you get the right fit, they can be more of a turn-on to some men than the scantiest piece of lingerie.

3. Jeans are versatile.
   There's almost no place that you can't wear jeans.

4. Jeans stand on their own.
   All you need to do is add a blazer to look finished.

Coats

I hope that everyone pays attention to their outerwear. It is one of the first things people see. Outerwear can be the core of a wardrobe. Don't skimp in this department. Don't wear an old torn coat if you can afford to change to a newer, fresher version. The current selection of cuts, colours and fabrics means that there is the perfect coat waiting out there for you.

Look for a Good Cut

You need enough room in the shoulder, sleeves and torso. You should be able to fit a heavy sweater or blazer comfortably underneath.

Durability

Look for sturdy lining. You'll find that the combination of rayon-acetate lasts the longest. Check to see that the lining is anchored at appropriate locations. It should be attached at the cuffs, armholes and hem.

Always in Style

Peacoat

Wrap coat

Princess shape

Reefer

Military coat

Double-breasted

Traditional camel

Proper Length

Where do you most like to wear your hemlines? Make sure your coat covers the length you are most apt to wear. Best bet? Pick a coat that almost sweeps to the ankles. You can wear this coat with dignity no matter what you have on underneath.

Casual Chic

Casual chic, otherwise known as 'weekend wear', is an easy and fun way to dress. Most days we are given the challenge of coming up with this look. The key is to look like you arrived at your look with little or no effort.

What's Not Casually Chic

Sweat pants and tops

Anything too matched

Clothes that are uncomfortable

Anything overly tailored

Grunge

Little girl looks

Rips and tears

Stained clothing

Laddered tights

Fallen hems

Worn-down shoes

Polyester

Too much jewellery

Too much perfume

Excessive makeup

Ill-fitting clothing

Un-ironed clothing

Lines or bulges under clothing

Trousers that are too short

Trousers that hang over shoes

Tights that are darker than shoes (in clothing other than jeans)

Heels with casual clothing

Stirrups showing under shoes

Athletic shoes

Wedgies

Anything transparent

Swimwear

Primal Fear

I have heard more primal screaming coming out of dressing rooms at swimsuit time than at any other time of the year. It doesn't matter what size you are or what age. Trying on swimwear has to rate right up there with the stirrups in gynaecologists' surgeries. I'm not saying that purchasing a swimsuit will ever be fun . . . fun . . . fun, but I can make it a little less painful for you.

Rule No. 1 – Go Up a Size

This is not what most women want to hear, but because swimsuits are made of less fabric than other garments, they tend to run a bit smaller than regular street clothing. A size twelve suit will be very snug on a woman who wears a size twelve dress, but will be perfect on a woman who wears a size ten. If you insist on trying on your regular size, make certain that you can bend, stretch, sit, etc., without any discomfort or riding up.

Rule No. 2 – Look at Labels

Thank the designer gods for finally listening to us. They have developed swimwear that actually gives the illusion of your having lost 5 kilos (10 pounds). You'll see the features written right on the label. Usually these suits are called *minimizers*. Again, try them on, because you may find them quite confining. It's nice to be tucked in, but who wants to feel like they're wearing a girdle on the beach?

Rule No. 3 – Don't Be Afraid of Colour

There is no reason to stick to black or navy if you're trying to give the illusion of slimness. Although darker colours do slim the body, vibrant shades like purple, magenta, maroon and green also serve this purpose. You can effectively use colour to accentuate the positive, while hiding any negatives. For instance, if you want to show off a terrific bosom, choose a bright colour in the bodice area with a darker bottom. Don't be afraid of lines in the fabric. Vertical lines can be especially flattering, as can geometric shapes and polka dots, because people's eyes never rest on a specific body area. Patterns keep the eyes moving.

Caring for Your Swimsuit

Hand wash after every wearing.

Do not put your suit in the dryer.

Always dry your swimsuit thoroughly before packing away.

Try not to get any lotions or sunscreens on your suit.

If you do get any lotion on your suit, use shampoo to sponge it off.

Working Style

Dressing for Success

We all know about dressing for corporate climbing and how the image that you present at work can enhance your chances of promotion and/or a salary increase. But that's not all there is to that story. Just putting on any structured suit will no longer do. The suit you choose to wear sends out a distinct message. The trick to buying a career suit is to find that fine balance between fitting in as a team member and sacrificing individuality. Many companies now realize that creative dressers are more open to new ideas than those who dress conservatively. How do you find the style that's right for you without being too risky? One that suits your body shape? Here are the secrets of a successful working wardrobe.

Choose a Style That Flatters Your Body Type

Triangle: Keep your jacket simple, yet slightly curvy.

Straight: Give the illusion of a slimmer waist with a light-coloured, loosely tailored jacket. Wear it over a fitted dark top and a belt.

Pear: Choose jackets with small, soft shoulder pads to give you more shape on top. Stay away from double-breasted jackets so that you don't add bulk to your hips.

Hour-glass: Sharp, masculine tailoring is not for you. Go for soft shapes and fabrics. You can get away with a knee-length pencil skirt or well tailored trousers.

Tips

1. The higher the quality, the better your suit will look in six months.

2. Buy a suit in a medium-weight fabric for year-round wear.

3. A neutral colour will provide more flexibility to mix and match with other clothes in your wardrobe.

4. Single-breasted jackets are more slimming.

5. Vertical stripes make you look taller and slimmer.

How to Wear Trousers

Trousers are now a very important part of the fashion scene. A good fit is a must when it comes to style.

Traditional

A flat-front straight-leg style is the most flattering for every body.

Petite

Choose high-waisted styles to give off the illusion of a longer leg.

Thin

Pleated trousers (menswear) creates a curvier leg.

Full Tummy

Softly draped trousers fall gracefully on the body.

Shopping Secrets

Try It On!

Make sure you look great from all angles of the mirror.

Stick to a List!

Stay with the pieces that will fill out your wardrobe, no matter how great a 'deal' some garment seems, or how trendy it is.

Don't Wait Until the Last Minute to Shop!

Never shop the day before an event. You are bound to make a big mistake. Of course, those last-minute events do occasionally occur. Just be prepared with a basic outfit that needs only a little accessorizing.

Be Very Careful of Sales!

It's only a good buy if you would pay full price for it.

Always Dress Well and Wear Make-up!

This is so important, because if you have no make-up on, everything looks horrible. If you're not well dressed, even the lowest of the low looks better than what you have on.

Shop Alone!

Well-meaning friends can talk you into a less than flattering look (the 'go ahead, you deserve it' routine), and salespeople can be just plain annoying. When one of them starts following you around the shop, simply explain that you need to be alone to sort through your wardrobe needs. It works every time!

Do's and Don'ts

Do...

Start your shopping trip in your own wardrobe.

Wear colour near your face.

Raid your man's wardrobe.

Be careful what you wear under your clothing.

Wear white in winter. It's called *winter white*.

Buy for the Body You Have

'It would look great if I just lost five pounds.'
How many of those 'promises' do you have
sitting in your wardrobe? By the time you've
lost the weight, that adorable outfit will be
unadorably out of fashion.

Add a trendy touch to each season's wardrobe.

Shop in second-hand designer shops.

Keep a core of five or six basics in your wardrobe.

Pick out two or three colours and plan your wardrobe around them.

Develop a theme for your wardrobe.

Purchase items that can be worn in any season.

Don't . . .

Be afraid to split up outfits.

Overaccessorize.

Try to hide figure flaws in oversized clothing.

Wear tops that display your favourite beer, cause, pet, your availability, etc.

Wear a full jacket with a full skirt.

Use more than two colours in an outfit.

Wear linen in winter.

Fix any part of your body in public.

Overspend on an item that you don't just love.

Send the wrong message with your clothing.

Keep your clothes so simple that you fade into the woodwork.

Purchase clothing that requires constant maintenance.

Chapter Eight
GLAMOUR

How to Go from Day to Evening

Situation No. 1

The phone rings. That invitation comes. You are invited to that special event, but there's a real problem. There will be no time to change into evening attire.

Situation No. 2

The office party is upon us, and we need to look good in a hurry!

Solution No. 1

Wear a basic black dress, basic skirt and top, or well-cut trouser outfit. Carry a few well-chosen accessories and stronger make-up colours.

Solution No. 2

A classic white shirt can go right into evening with a frilly skirt and diamanté accessories.

Solution No. 3

A well-cut pair of trousers can take on a new life with a sequined T-shirt.

Solution No. 4

A black round-neck sweater can be belted with a diamanté

or petersham belt and added to a satin skirt for last-minute panache.

Solution No. 5

A basic suit jacket can go into the evening when paired with satin or lace trousers.

Solution No. 6

Take a regular day suit and remove the blouse under the jacket. Extra skin is appropriate for the evening hours. If you're feeling just too under-dressed, then add a little lace hanky at the bodice.

What Does That Invitation Mean?

The invitation came in the post today, and you haven't a clue what to wear. You've never been to this kind of event, and you won't know a soul there. Just what does that invitation mean?

The invitation says 'Informal'

If the invitation is printed or engraved (as opposed to a handwritten one from a friend), 'informal' does not mean jeans! Men wear lounge suits, and women wear something smart but not too dressy. Depending on the hour, the venue and the occasion, you could wear anything from a classic suit with a silk blouse to the dependable little black dress to an evening trouser suit. Jewellery and other accessories should be relatively understated; and shoes with heels are preferable to flats.

The invitation says 'Black Tie'

Here, too, a wide range of outfits can be worn – anything from a cocktail dress to a long dress. If it's a dinner or an official function, the style should be fairly covered up; for a dance you can bare more skin. Flowing evening trousers are a stylish option, perhaps with a glitzy top.

The invitation says 'White Tie'

This is the time to go all-out for glamour. Your best ball-gown, your most splendid jewellery and even long white gloves can be worn. (Bracelets are worn under the gloves, which are kept on for drinking, removed for eating.) You can also indulge in extra make-up for these grand occasions.

Help! It's a Black Tie!

When black tie is required, think formal but understated. It's a different look from white tie, in that there is more flexibility. You can show up in a long dress, but a well-fitted dress and jacket would be just as acceptable. A satin dress or formal trouser suit is perfectly fine.

Weddings

Weddings held in the daytime normally call for morning dress for men – striped grey or black trousers, waistcoat and black tailcoat. Women are correspondingly elegant, in smart dresses or suits, usually with a hat (although many younger women go hatless now). A trouser suit can be worn, but it should be in a dressy fabric. Colour has long been a contentious issue. Black, once frowned on because of its funereal associations, has become acceptable, though navy is a better alternative. Some etiquette experts even allow white, but I say don't wear it! Choose another pale shade, if pale is what you fancy, to show some respect for the bride.

Avoid anything sparkly, like sequins, unless the wedding is held in the evening.

Quick Glamour

It shouldn't take all day to look extra-special. Here are some quick tips for that glamorous look.

Hair

Instant Glamour

To give hair fullness and bounce, lift dry hair at the roots with a round brush. Pull it taut, and squirt with hair spray. Then blow-dry hair on the warm setting at high strength. Using the warm setting makes hair flexible, and allows you to restyle it. For even more fullness, bend forwards, so that head is tilted down when drying. Finish styling as usual.

Sparkling, Shining Hair

Give your hair a dazzling, party-perfect finish by squirting it with a shine spray. There are several good ones on the market. Apply shine through dry hair, then brush through for even distribution.

Eyes

Fast Frames

To give the eye definition and mystery, brush brows up to accentuate the arch. Set it with a toothbrush sprayed with hair spray. Finish off by adding a bit of white shadow under the brow. If necessary, before spraying, pencil along the natural arch.

Mystery Eyes

The smoky eye is the perfect look for 'after five'. Take a black pencil or liquid liner, and line both above and below the eye. Soften the look, and secure it by running over the lines with lighter shadow.

Take the Plunge!

Little strappy, low-cut dresses put your flesh on display! Make sure it's blemish-free by gently exfoliating to lift off dead skin, even out skin tone and discourage blemishes. Toners will help keep oiliness under control, but be certain to wipe off residue with witch hazel or lemon.

If you do have blemished skin, don't panic! Take a water-resistant concealer and pat it over the area until it blends with the surrounding area. A quick pat of powder will set it. If you have lines, smooth a firming face gel over the area (be sure to check the breast area).

Keep skin soft and silky by spraying on body oils that both scent and polish shoulders, breasts and upper arms. Here's a way to boost the sheen. Just mix a touch of gold powder with the oil in the palms of your hands, then smooth it on.

Add a little bronzing powder into the cleavage, but be sure to blend well.

The Evening Bag

There are two schools of thought when it comes to evening bags. There's the person who carries as little as possible, and then there's the person who can't go out for the evening without throwing in the kitchen sink. There are guidelines for both; just plan ahead!

The Minimalist

Money?
Enough cash to hail a cab

Cosmetics?
A lipstick and compact

Anything Else?
Breath mints
A comb
Maybe a hanky
Key

The Pack Rat

Money?
Not only a substantial amount of money (up to £50), but a credit card (or two)

Cosmetics?
Lipstick, foundation, blush, mascara and liner
Adhesive to re-apply false eyelashes

Anything Else?
Cellular phone
Condom
Key

Chapter Nine
THE FINISHING TOUCH

Didn't You Know?

Accessories Make the Woman

Show me a well-dressed woman, and I'll show you someone who knows the fine art of accessorizing. Accessories
are the finishing touch that gives us our individuality and
shows us just how far we can go with a little imagination.
It is the least expensive way to extend a wardrobe and the
first evidence of good taste. Here's what I consider to be
the most important accessories in any woman's wardrobe.

The Handbag

You thought shoes were the most important accessory in
a woman's wardrobe? Wrong! It's your handbag. It's at eye
level after all! The perfect handbag is never larger than 25
x 33cm (10 x 13in). Although it's not necessary to match
a handbag to every outfit, there should be some kind of
co-ordination effort. Always choose the best handbag you
can possibly afford. To be well groomed, it is absolutely
essential for you to include the following items:

Lipstick (doubles as blush)

Compact (choose dual finish)

Notebook with pen

Wallet

Breath mints

Comb or brush

Neutral eye shadow (doubles as lip powder)

Eyeliner

Tissues

This is a 'must have' list. Of course, if there's room add these:

Mini pill box with supplies

Sewing kit

Mascara

Hair 'scrunchy'

Nail file

While on the Go

Timesavers

Carry your make-up in a see-through pencil case. It will eliminate wasted time rummaging through your entire bag.

Always carry a mirror in your bag.

Don't ever carry loose powder!

If you must choose one colour, pick a black bag, which will go with about everything!

Be sure that the handles fit neatly over your shoulder before purchasing your bag. The kind you carry in your hand, while attractive, is impractical.

Shoes

I have never had a problem convincing women of the importance of shoes. It's the men who wear their shoes forever, and get them continually resoled as though they're desperate to keep an old friend. It's the type of shoe that women choose that can make or break a totally finished look. Also, the care they give their shoes is crucial in giving that all-important final, finishing touch. Scuffed heels, sloppy fit and salt marks can be fixed in moments. And they should be!

Heels

Allow me to share an old model's trick with you. A lot of modelling is not as glamorous as you may have been led to believe. There are levels of modelling that include promotion work, trade shows and other similar assignments. It means that these beautiful models must remain on their feet, in high heels, looking glamorous for hours at a time.

How do they do it without collapsing? The secret is to go up one full size from your regular shoe size. If you're a size 8 in a loafer, then you would take a size 9 in an 8cm (3in) heel. This allows for the inevitable swelling that takes place during the day. For those who need to look 'together' and polished throughout a long and tedious work day, heels from 2.5 to 5cm (1¹/₂ to 2 in) high are the most comfortable.

Fabric

If you can afford the rich buttery leather of a designer shoe, your benefits include comfort and flexibility. If it's completely out of your price range, try at least to stay away from man-made materials. They don't last very long, and they are low on the comfort scale. It's impossible for a foot to breathe in vinyl or plastic.

Shoes that are tight when you are being fitted never can become comfortable. The one exception is suede, which has a bit more stretchability.

Perhaps you have those shoes that you just couldn't resist, and you hoped would stretch out, sitting in your closet. Try this: Wet the inside of the shoes with an equal amount of water and alcohol. Stuff the shoes with newspaper, and leave them out to dry overnight. This just might make them wearable.

What Else to Watch Out For

Back Height and Heel Pinch

Hold backs together to check that they are equal height. Then put each shoe down to make sure that they sit flat.

Toe Spring

You should be able to slip a pencil under the front of the shoe.

Synthetics/Leather

On the shoe it should state clearly what the shoe is made of.

Top Line

Look at the inside of the heel to check that the shoe's outside rim is straight.

Top Stitching

This should be straight and well-machined. If it's uneven, the shoe is poorly made.

Sole Bonding

If you can pull the sole away, they haven't used the right adhesive. Under the innersole, you should have a little cushion for comfort.

Heel Attachment

If you run your finger around the innersole and feel bumps, the wrong kind of nail has been used.

Sandals

1. Consider what you'll be wearing with your sandals, and purchase the simplest pair.
2. If you tend to wear patterns, choose black or white sandals.
3. Buy the right size. Your heels and toes should not hang over the edges of the sandals. Make sure that the strappy parts of the sandals aren't too tight or flimsy.

Stitched Sole

A leather sole should be stitched, or welted, to the upper. A channel is cut into the sole, the shoe is stitched together, and then the channel is put back to hide the stitching. You should clearly see the welt mark running all around the sole. Leather soles are better than resin.

Hosiery

The purpose of everything I share with you is meant to simplify your life, not complicate it. That is why I refuse to go into a long soliloquy on what per cent of nylon versus Lycra you should have in your tights for longevity. Here are the rules. Follow them, and you'll get value for your money.

Do ...

Wear black opaque stockings or tights. They are the most practical and slimming hosiery you'll ever own.

Match your shoes and tights when you can. This is a very appealing and slimming look.

Hand wash your tights in a mild detergent.

Wear tights with reinforced toes when not wearing open-toed shoes.

Stock up on your favourite tights when they go on sale.

Give your tights a quick spray of hair lacquer to resist runs.

Throw out snagged tights. If you can't bear to do this, wear them only under trousers.

Sunglasses

Another important finishing touch to any woman's wardrobe is her sunglasses. The general rule is to choose a frame that complements your facial structure.

Long Narrow Face

Looks best in wraparound, oval frames.

Round Face

Looks best in square glasses.

Square Face

Looks best in round frames.

Long Nose

Stay away from aviator styles.

Jewellery at Work

In the office, jewellery can give ordinary work clothes out-standing style. It can add sparkle and fun to an otherwise serious environment. Keep jewellery understated in the workplace. Bracelets shouldn't get in the way of writing or typing. One or two conversation brooches are a statement. Several brooches become a walking jewellery chest. Don't be afraid to show your personal style at work. The right jewellery can make whatever you wear more sophisticated and noteworthy.

Jewellery Do's and Don'ts

Do...

Mix metals.

Mix pearls with metals.

Pile on several chains together (this look was invented by Coco Chanel).

Bring daytime into evening with crystal jewellery.

Have fun with your jewellery.

Combine chokers with long strands.

Use bracelets to create cuffs.

Add brooches to your handbags, lapels and pockets.

Use brooches as icebreakers at an event where you're not known.

Use a brooch as a necklace enhancer to change a look.

Tack down a scarf with a coordinating brooch.

Dress up denim with jewellery.

Soften the look of leather with pearls.

Use power jewellery for evening.

Bring a trouser suit into evening with crystal pieces.

Feel free to knot, double and treble pearls.

Wear two chokers at once (a wonderful frame for the face).

Mix real gems with fake.

Mix matt and shiny materials.

Don't...

Wear dangle jewellery at work.

Wear perfume near pearl (the oil will eat away the coating).

Wear jewellery in your nose.

Wear big earrings AND a big necklace.

Wear a lot of crystal or other glittery jewellery during the day.

Wear white jewellery with white clothing.

Wear a daytime watch with evening attire.

Put a dainty ring on a large hand.

Be afraid to wear heirlooms.

Think of costume jewellery as tacky.

Wear pendants longer than the belt line.

115

THE WORLD'S BEST-KEPT BEAUTY SECRETS

Forget to co-ordinate your jewellery with your belt (both are important accessories).

Be afraid to wear a brooch or two on your shoulder to pick up your posture.

Wear two watches at once, even if it's a pendant watch and bracelet watch.

Be afraid to shop in flea markets for jewellery bargains.

Forget to clean your jewellery weekly.

Secrets of Scarves

A scarf can double as a head wrap.

Use a scarf as a colourful belt.

If you've got a neat little waist, tie a large scarf around it for a Spanish look.

A simple square scarf is a provocative face flatterer.

A scarf makes a wild necktie.

Fill in a suit with a scarf used as an ascot.

Tie a scarf on a handbag to totally co-ordinate your outfit.

A small scarf makes a delightful wrist band.

A rolled scarf is a necklace.

Any hat looks more festive with the addition of a scarf.

Purchase silk fabric and make your own scarf.

Wear your scarf as a bow tie.

Belts

Chain Belts

Wear chain belts draped loosely around the hips. Women with larger waists can easily wear belts without accentuating their flaws.

Hipster Belts

Be careful to leave a bit of slack when wearing this type of belt. Pulling this type of belt too tightly will cause the fabric to bunch.

Colours

Wearing a belt in the same tone as a skirt or trousers is more slimming.

Chapter Ten

BARGAINS

Beauty on a Budget

It's time to take charge of your beauty and your budget. Do you truly believe that you can't look good and stay solvent? Then this chapter will change the way you approach your beauty purchases. Once you take just a little bit of extra time to read labels and explore new stockists, you will be amazed at just how much you can save. Many of the same name brands, cosmetic counter items you've been tied to for years, contain the same ingredients as the chemists' own brands or generic versions.

Discounts Galore

More and more consumer goods are becoming available at a discount, and this includes fashions and even some cosmetics. Here are just a few of the many places where you can find genuine bargains.

The Address/Designer Exchange
3 Royal Exchange Court
Glasgow G1 3DB
tel: 0141 221 6898

Famous labels from Armani to Jaeger to Versace, at about one-third the original price, are offered here, along with nearly-new outfits, many worn by celebrities.

The British Designer Sale for Women
42 York Mansions
Prince of Wales Drive
London SW11 4BP
tel: 0171 228 5314

For the past twenty years this organisation has been offering designer clothes at huge discounts – five times a year for women, twice a year for men – now at the Chelsea Town Hall. Two other sales a year are held in Edinburgh. Sales are open to current members only (for current fee, contact the organization), but the discounts, which range from 50 to 80 per cent off the original price, recoup this investment many times over.

The Designer Warehouse Sales
The Worx
45 Balfe Street
London N1 3DF
tel: 0171 704 1064

Six sales a year offer women's clothing and accessories by designer names such as Nicole Farhi, Dolce & Gabbana, Workers for Freedom and Osprey at one-third off the original price. Join the mailing list to be kept informed of sale dates. There is a modest admission charge.

Great Western Designer Outlet Village
Kemble Drive
Rodbourne
Swindon SN2 2DY
tel: 01793 507600

119

This 108-unit shopping complex includes many shops selling famous-name clothing, lingerie and accessories, such as Christian Lacroix, Windsmoor, Jane Shilton and Pied à Terre, at reductions of between 30 and 70 per cent. Most are perfect (overstocks from previous seasons); some are seconds.

Jackson's Landing Factory Shops
The Highlight
Hartlepool Marina
Hartlepool
Cleveland TS24 0XN
tel: 01429 866 9890

In this development, which includes a fashion department store and twenty-one factory outlets, you'll find clothing and accessories by the likes of Jasper Conran, Calvin Klein, Louis Feraud, Planet and Warners at substantial discounts.

Next to Nothing
Unit 11
Waterglade Centre
London W5 2ND
tel: 0181 567 2747

104 Corporation Street
Birmingham
West Midlands B2 6XS
tel: 0121 233 0022

Clothing from the Next chain is offered here at 50 to 75 per cent less than the original prices. Most items are ex-sale stock, with further reductions.

TK MAXX

Many shops throughout Britain; for addresses telephone:

Banbury: 01295 277022
Belfast: 01232 331151
Bournemouth: 01202 316367
Bristol: 0117 930 4404
Croydon: 0181 686 9753
Dudley: 01384 77878
Glasgow: 0141 331 0411
Hanley: 01782 207509
Harrogate: 01423 536636
Hull: 01482 223202
Leicester: 0116 251 0155
Liverpool: 0151 708 9919
Newcastle: 0191 261 0404
Preston: 01772 253220
Reading: 01734 511117
Southampton: 01703 631600
Sutton: 0181 770 7796
Woking: 01483 771660

This American retailer offers famous-label clothing, shoes, lingerie, fragrance and cosmetics, among other goods, at prices between 20 and 60 per cent less than you'll find in high-street shops. New stock (guaranteed to be the real thing) is constantly arriving.

Yves Rocher Cosmetics
Yves Rocher Ltd.
Freepost
664 Victoria Road
South Ruislip
Middlesex HA4 0BR
tel: 0181 845 1222
fax: 0181 845 1023

They run introductory offers of their cosmetics at considerable reductions, featured in fashion and general-interest magazines. (Products are not tested on animals.)

Looks That Won't Kill (Your Budget, That Is)

A budget-based beauty regime doesn't mean losing out on quality, or the 'feel good' factor. Yes, you can look like a class act without spending a fortune, if you know which products work. Here's a list that will leave you and your bank balance looking just fine.

Cleansers

Since they all perform the same task, why spend a fortune on a product that is on the skin only for a few seconds? Get a cheap cream-based cleanser if you have dry skin, or a gel-based cleanser for oily skin. Better yet, simply wash your face with a little milk. It's much cheaper, and better for your skin because it contains lactic acid.

Acquaeous cream, a very effective cleanser, can be obtained from pharmaceutical counters at a little over £2 for a huge 500g (17³/₄oz) pot. You tissue it off, then rinse. The cream can also be used as a moisturizer.

Toners

Spending any money at all on a toner is a big waste when, for less than 20p, the ultimate toner is readily available. A lemon is the best way to restore the pH balance. Need something that does not carry a code? A little witch hazel will do just fine!

Moisturizers

Purchase an inexpensive moisturizer at the chemist. Don't spend even a few pence more for any enrichments. Alternate between adding a vitamin A capsule in the morning and a vitamin E capsule at night. This is what

Hair

The best bargain for your hair is a good cut.

If possible, pay extra for a top-of-the-line stylist

(sometimes called a master stylist). More

technically advanced hair cuts will last longer

(up to eight weeks depending on the length). Save

money by using chalk to touch up telltale roots.

you're hearing all the hype about. It's pretty much the same formula that they expect you to spend £25 or £30 for. Add your own vitamins, and get a more powerful effect. Don't spend too much more for sunscreen protection. You can always add your own base of sunscreen before moisturizing.

Cosmetics

Try to find as many cosmetics as possible that perform two or more jobs. For years models have been using lipstick as blush, and eye shadow to seal and powder lips. You can also use eye pencil as lip pencil. Unfortunately, lip pencils contain ingredients that cannot be used in the eye area. Create gentle contouring on the cheeks and sides of the nose with a neutral lip pencil.

Organize your cosmetics in an old-fashioned tackle box purchased from a shop selling fishing supplies.

Shampoos

There are very good brands available in drugstores. L'Oréal, Clairol and others offer excellent value along with their good names. Don't forget to enhance your shampoos with vodka (for shine) and vinegar (to remove residue). Rely on the conditioners you can easily make from scratch (refer to Chapter Three).

Facials

Here's the facial that costs nothing yet is highly beneficial. Steam your face by bending over a bowl of boiling water with your favourite herbal tea.

Fade dark circles under your eyes by placing the same cold tea bags over your eyes for about ten minutes.

Cook two carrots until soft, then mash. Apply to your face, and let harden. This vitamin A mask is beneficial and refreshing!

Facial Toning

Tone up your facial muscles with water. Fill up your mouth with as much water as possible. Hold it there for as long as you can. Allow the water pressure to do all the work for you.

Jut out your lower jaw. Gently raise your chin towards your nose, stretching your neck muscles. Then lower your chin back down to the starting position. Do this in the car, while talking on the phone, etc. This exercise will prevent 'turkey jowl'.

Open your eyes (as in a surprised expression) and try to reach your forehead. Do this several times.

Free Advice

Some British department stores now offer a personal shopping service. It won't cost you anything, and you'll get the unbiased opinion that you can't get from friends, commissioned salespeople or your partner. Don't bother to spend money on a professional image consultant. Every consultant I have ever interviewed uses silly formulas for colours, matching fabrics and other structured stuff that nobody has time for. Plus, you'll hear a different opinion from each image consultant you meet. Can't get out to a shop? Some mail-order catalogues offer free advice over the phone. Be sure you have the company's catalogue with you.

Home Treatments

Colour and perfume your own Epsom salts for a delightful bathtime experience. Find salts in any chemists. Store them in a big glass jar with a lid. Sprinkle in a few drops of food colouring, close the jar and shake it vigorously until the colour is evenly distributed. Then pour it out onto a baking tray, and let it dry. You can speed things by placing it in a warm oven for a half an hour if you prefer. Perfume your salts with a little perfume oil. Just add a few drops of your favourite fragrance, and shake again until there aren't any clumpy bits. You can add sea salt and bicarbonate of soda to give it a different texture. Add a metal scoop, and you have your very own bath treatment.

To combat dryness, add a cup of oatmeal and a tablespoon of avocado oil to a warm bath. Soak for at least 15 minutes.

While you're relaxing in the tub, increase the moisturizing effect by mashing two strawberries with two teaspoons of yoghurt. Leave it on your face for 15 minutes. If you have any left over, rub it over the gum area to promote healthy gums.

Remove excess oils from your face by mashing a tablespoon of pineapple and applying it to your face for 15 minutes then rinsing.

After shaving legs, rub a slice of cucumber over them. Cleopatra used to have her legendary skin rubbed with cooked cucumber peelings.

Tips

Don't buy an expensive cosmetic bag. A plastic pencil case is just the right size and transparent, to make finding things a snap.

To extend the life of nail varnish, clean the top of the bottle with a tissue after applying. Polish buildup allows air into the bottle, and the product will evaporate.

Almond oil will stop acrylic nails from dehydrating and coming away from the nail plate.

Save on accessories by shopping in girls' and teens' areas of department stores. You can save on such things as hair accessories, costume jewellery, handbags and scarves.

Use hair spray to stop static cling.

Get the most out of your fragrance by applying it only to pulse point areas. A lot of perfume is wasted by spraying it into the air.

Save leftover lipstick, and pack it down in a small paint box or pill box.

File only the tips of your nails and your manicure will last longer.

Massage leftover hair conditioner into your cuticles.

Explore charity shops when you have a large block of time. Since this type of shops doesn't have to worry much about cash flow, you'll find ten times the merchandise that you would find in a boutique. It may take patience and time, but the rewards are unending for the diligent bargain hunter.

Use oversized, outdated earrings to glamorize a pair of plain pumps.

Add your own buttons to a pair of gloves for a designer look.

Add tassels to scarves for a rich style.

Cut buttons off old clothing, and recycle them for other clothes.

Witch hazel makes a great hair degreaser for dry shampooing.

Check to see if your health insurance company will pay for sunscreen.

Shop in hardware stores for great buys on chains for pendants and belts.

Use floor wax to protect shoes and handbags and keep them shiny.

Have a clothing swap with friends, and see how great your shopping mistakes can look on someone else.

Use eye shadow as liner by wetting it down and applying with a fine brush.

Mix your own colours by combining lipsticks and eye shadows.

Shop in men's and boys' departments for great buys in sweaters, shirts and workout clothing.

Go through your own cupboards once a month and discard any redundant items.

Use less of products than is recommended on the packaging. Many manufacturers tell you to use more, so that you'll run out faster.

Use baby oil instead of make-up remover.

Shopping Sales

Twice a year, in late June/early July and in late December/early January, shops offer the previous season's leftover merchandise at substantial reductions. This is your chance to pick up that stunning silk blouse you were coveting, or those frivolous shoes that weren't quite worth the original price, at a substantial saving. What's more, a lot of retailers now offer mid-season reductions, too – to get rid of slow-moving items and to lure shoppers into the store at times when business is a little slack. The only trouble with sales is that one is often tempted to buy something just because it's reduced. If it isn't something you'd want to buy at full price, it isn't really a bargain.

Chapter Eleven
ANTI-AGEING

Simple Ways to Resist Ageing

By cutting down or avoiding the following, you can help your skin to look younger a lot longer.

The Sun

It's the number-one reason why our skin ages. Wear sunscreen at all times, and don't forget protective clothing. Don't forget that the scalp also needs to be protected from the sun.

Smoking

Early wrinkling occurs due to reduced levels of the oxygen needed to keep skin healthy. Smoking is the prime source of oxygen deprivation. If you are in the process of quitting, drink lots of water.

Alcohol

In excess, alcohol dehydrates the body and robs it of vitamins that keep skin both healthy and glowing. If possible, always follow an alcoholic drink with a chaser of iced water.

Improper Nutrition

The modern-day use of convenience foods encourages the formation of free radicals. These foods are high in processed fats and oils. Protection of the skin is possible by eating foods rich in vitamins A, C and E. Fresh fruits and vegetables are particularly good for keeping the skin youthful. Supplementation may be necessary if you're not getting these nutrients in your foods.

Purchases Every Ageing Beauty Must Make

Three-Way Mirror

Especially after age forty, you must be certain you look as good going as you do coming. Unfortunately, some of the first signs of ageing come from behind.

Magnifying Mirror

There are things happening to your face and body, that the ageing eye may not see. A three- to-five-times magnification mirror will help you to check on such exciting agers as brown spots, facial hair and wrinkles.

The Right Magazines and Literature

There is a wealth of magazines and self-help books geared for women who are no longer twenty nor have any wish to go back to that time in their lives. You need the magazine that tells you that it is perfectly acceptable to forgo the grunge and rubber looks for something that may be a bit more appropriate to the 'classic' beauty.

A Jump Rope

For women who are unable to get into a full exercise programme, skipping rope tones arm and leg muscles while building cardiovascular endurance. Increased heart and lung performance will result in increased blood flow to the skin's surface. A good walk will do, a good run is better, but do something at least three times a week. This will also keep cellulite and varicose veins from creeping in.

Bronzing Powder

Never leave home without the youthful look of a tan. Now you can do it safely. There is nothing short of plastic surgery that looks more rested. There's not one factor that will age you faster than the natural way of getting one. Use bronzing powder liberally over the face, décolletage and neck. It will take the years off quickly and efficiently.

Stress

A constant menu of stress causes the skin to become sensitive and prone to blemishes. Regular exercise and meditation will help diffuse its effects. Lying on a bed with your head hanging down off the side is a super de-stresser.

Plastic Surgery

Once considered extreme, cosmetic surgery is now being done on women and men of all incomes and ages. If you are considering plastic surgery, there are a few things that you need to know before searching out a plastic surgeon. If you've been looking in the mirror, pushing this, pulling that, and you're just tired of it, then you may feel that it's time. With all the new procedures available to you today, there's no reason to be afraid; just be informed. Here's an idea of what you're in for.

Eyelid Surgery

The cost for an eye lift is in the area of £1,800 to £2,800, depending on the extent of the surgery. (This includes an overnight stay in hospital.) The recovery period is about two weeks, after which you'll be able to hide the scarring with cosmetics. The eyes are often the first feature to show ageing. The skin loses elasticity, and there is a weakening of muscle. Fat pushes forward to shroud the eye.

Facelift

A complete facelift (excluding the eyes) costs about £3,700, including two nights in hospital.

Liposuction

Prices for this operation vary enormously, depending on how much fat you want to remove from the body. The most common target areas are the thighs, saddle bags (upper thighs), inside the knees and the neck.

Chemical Face Peel

This procedure runs the range depending on the strength of the peel. Please keep in mind that a peel is for wrinkling only. It won't help with the loss of elasticity. Find a surgeon who specializes in peeling or laser surgery for the best result.

Be Advised:

Check out 'before' and 'after' pictures of actual results.

Don't rely too much on computer imaging. Surgeons work on real people, not on machines.

Check to see that your surgeon is board certified.

Find a surgeon who will listen to your overall concerns.

Disregard anyone who promises you miracles.

Don't Stop Changing

Don't become a caricature of what you were at 20 or 30. Women who are guilty of this tend to wear the look that they had when they felt their most attractive. You've seen these women on the street wearing that Farrah Fawcett hairdo. They're still sporting that beehive hairdo or that Elizabeth Taylor 'Cleopatra' eye makeup. Their foundation looks like they laid it on with a spatula.

Anti-Ageing Rule No. 1

Update your make-up the way you update your wardrobe.

Anti-Ageing Rule No. 2

Age gracefully and you'll always remain youthful.

Chapter Twelve
TRAVEL

How to Pack

Packing is an art. You can be born with a gift for it. Do it enough, and you'll become an expert at it. It requires discipline, creativity and a great deal of patience.

Luggage

The ideal travel wardrobe is like a well-planned itinerary. It will provide for everything that you need. Whether you need it for a week or a big weekend, you want to include just what you'll wear and nothing more. You'll need to choose items that work with each other. Choose luggage that is both light and durable. Some luggage is heavy before anything is packed in it. This is the last luggage you would ever want to choose. Stay away from it. Today's luggage is made from modern materials that weigh next to nothing and perform their job beautifully and durably. Also avoid luggage that has no bend or give to it.

Colours

This area requires a good deal of restraint, but try to stick to two colours when packing. For instance, black and ivory are two colours that work well when travelling. You'll add one more colour for dimension and accenting. If you're choosing black and ivory, choose red for a dash of pizzazz.

Clothes

Take those few key pieces (trousers, shorts, skirt, jacket) according to the climate you are visiting, and let your accessories carry you through. Lay everything out on the bed and create different combinations before packing.

Packing

Bulky or heavy items should be placed at the very bottom and sides of the suitcase. This prevents them from falling down, and wrinkling clothing as soon as the suitcase is picked up. Fill shoes with socks and underwear, and slip them into plastic bags to protect your clothing. Place high heels with the heel towards the middle, so that they won't ruin your luggage. Plastic bags are slippery, so you can pack a lot more. Perfume bottles should be placed inside shoes. Not only will this protect the bottle, but it also maintains the shape of the shoe.

Cosmetics

Try to find a compact beauty case. If you like to hang your cosmetics from the back of the bathroom door hook, choose a roll-type cosmetic bag. Fill your cosmetic bag with travel-sized items. You should be able to go to your local department store, and get sample sizes of just about every cosmetic you will need. Seal all toiletries in plastic bags.

Packing Tricks

Fold long, easily wrinkled fabrics around sturdier ones. For instance, pack your elegant silk jumpsuit around your jeans.

Jewellery

When packing jewellery, every smart traveller

makes use of some clever tricks. If you're

planning to bring some necklaces along,

just wrap them around a hair roller. Secure

them with an elastic band. They'll unroll

perfectly . . . with no more knots or tangles.

Don't pack anything you don't wear at home.

Pack a large scarf or two. You'll find this is one of the most useful travel items. You can wear it as a sarong, use it as a swimsuit cover, use it in place of a blouse to wear under suits and even use it to strategically cover stains.

Upon arrival at your hotel, unpack everything and hang any wrinkled garments in the bathroom or shower to steam away wrinkling. Always include a sewing kit, scissors and a clothes brush or sticky tape.

A hairdryer takes on another life when travelling. It's a quick dryer for tights, lingerie and small stains.

The plastic bags you've packed will be used at your destination for laundry and wet swimsuit storage.

137

Use a good-sized tote to carry onto the plane anything you consider a necessity. That usually includes eyeglasses or contact lens items, money, camera, medications, real jewellery, passport and reading materials.

Pack a foldaway bag for the souvenirs you won't be able to live without.

Bring a small address book for postcards and emergency phone numbers.

When travelling to a foreign country, always take a skirt. You never know whom you might offend by wearing trousers.

In the Air

Drink plenty of liquids to counteract the drying effects of 'canned' air.

Wear spectacles instead of contact lenses.

Pre-order a special meal (it will be fresher).

Grab a pillow and blanket upon boarding.

Bring a toothbrush and toothpaste for long flights.

Always wear something comfortable like an oversized sweater you can cuddle up in.

Don't drink more than one alcoholic drink. It's very dehydrating.

Bring slippers or slipper socks to keep your feet warm when you slip off your shoes.

Dress in layers so you can add or subtract as the temperature in the cabin changes.

Did You Know?

The air quality in economy is better than it is in first class. That's because more bodies mean more humidity.

Your shoes may not fit at the end of your flight. Your feet will swell considerably in the air, so be sure that your shoes are a bit roomy starting out. Or drink lots of water while in the air, and put your feet up as much as possible.

Your hair will become full of static during your flight. That's because of the dry air. Use a silicone-based defrizzer to coat it.

Epsom salts will relieve jet lag. After a flight, add 400g (15oz) of Epsom salts to your bath water. The magnesium chloride will draw out wastes and leave you feeling tranquil.

You can ask to have your mini-bar contents removed from your hotel room. You'll avoid temptation this way.

Special Destinations

Ski Vacations

Always wear a moisturizing sunscreen of at least 15 SPF.

Use powder-based foundation so that there will be no rub-off on your clothes.

To keep colour on your lips, line the entire lip with pencil and finish off with a lip balm.

Don't bother with blush. The outdoors will give you a natural glow.

A high ponytail or plaits will control long hair, and are perfectly acceptable on the slopes.

Avoid 'hat head' by wearing earmuffs or a headband.

Wearing a one-piece ski suit will be more slimming than wearing separates.

Lycra will also pare off the pounds.

Use extra conditioning treatments on your hair to avoid static from hats.

Sun Spots

Good sunglasses are essential for eye safety and protection against wrinkles.

Wear clothes with a built-in UV block. Pure silk, high shine polyester and towelling are sun blockers. Stay away from bleached cottons and crepes.

Stage your workout in the pool. The natural buoyancy causes the muscles to work harder, and it feels just great.

Use the beach's sand to exfoliate your skin. Rub it all over those rough spots.

Leave your hair conditioner on while in the sun. It acts like a heat cap.

Sprinkle talcum powder into shoes before wearing.

Wear cotton underclothing.

Stay cool with loose-fitting clothing and elasticated waistbands.

Chapter Thirteen
MAINTENANCE & ORGANIZATION

Protect Your Investments

After spending a small fortune on your wardrobe, shoes and accessories, it just doesn't make any sense not to keep your things in good repair. You'll end up keeping them longer and looking your best at a moment's notice. Remember, you never know when you'll need to head out the door in a hurry. You take care of your car, your kids and your home. Why won't you give yourself the same consideration? It doesn't take that long and it's well worth the effort. It's guaranteed to make life easier for you in the long run.

The Big Clean-up

Here's how to make your wardrobe more wearable.

1. Go through your closet and get rid of anything you haven't worn in two seasons.

2. Get rid of mistakes. If it doesn't have any place to go, give it one. Your local charity!

3. Toss out what doesn't fit. Face reality. It hurts more to look at that piece of clothing than it does to clear it out.

4. Make repairs. Chances are, the garment is not being utilized simply because it's not ready to go out.

5. Items you are absolutely forever attached to must be stored.

6. Hang clothes by category, outfit or possibilities.

Clothes Care

Check dry cleaning instructions. Throwing a delicate fabric into the washing machine will ruin its finish.

Invest in padded hangers. Wire hangers can leave shoulder marks or ridges.

Wrap hangers in tissue paper to support heavier clothing.

Keep leather and suede garments and shoes supple by treating them with a protective cream.

Iron inside out to avoid dulling the gleam of the fabric.

Remove lint from knits and woollens by shaving the surface with an electric razor or sweater shaver.

Treat shoes and bags with a stain repellent.

Wash or dry clean clothing before storing. Moths are less attracted to clean clothes.

Dry cleaning is the quickest way to freshen a tired garment.

When storing clothes, keep moths away by putting some dry bay leaves between layers in storage boxes and garment bags. Bay leaves won't leave the distasteful odour found in mothballs.

Jackets must be hung to keep their shape. Stuff arms with tissue paper or newspaper.

Always button and zip clothing to hang properly and to maintain space in your wardrobe.

Fold sweaters. Hanging them will cause them mysteriously to grow!

Apply a thin coat of clear nail varnish or nail hardener to pearl buttons to restore their lustre and make them more durable.

To remove deodorant stains, rub clothing with a little ammonia before laundering. For regular stains, mix three parts bicarbonate of soda to two parts vinegar.

Instead of buying expensive garment bags to protect your hanging clothes from fading, cover them with old pillowcases.

Perfume padded hangers to scent your clothing.

Get More Life Out of Your Clothing

Altering clothing gives them a new life. Long skirts can be shortened, wide trousers can be taken in and shoulder pads can easily be removed.

Shoes

Use an old-fashioned rubber to remove grime from suede and fabric shoes.

Use a soft cloth or brush (not wire) to loosen surface dirt.

A black felt-tip pen can colour in scuff marks.

Store your boots on boot trees. If you don't have room, stuff them as much as possible with newspaper.

Pull out the inner sole of a shoe or boot and let it air out periodically.

Never let shoes dry near a radiator or heating duct. Too much heat may crack the leather and shrink the skin.

Go easy on waterproofing and harsh chemical treatments. Some of the ones on the market today can do as much harm as good. Nikwax make a variety of good waterproofing products for shoes and clothing.

To remove salt stains from boots, dampen a sponge with white vinegar. Gently blot away marks.

To rid suede of water marks, brush against the grain. Allow it to dry. If it's a soft suede, fill with tissue or newspaper to ensure the integrity of the shape.

Erase dark marks from pale leather by dabbing with nail varnish remover.

Blot grease stains with a paper towel. Follow up by massaging with talcum powder for five minutes. Brush away with a soft brush.

Clean patent leather with a glass cleaner. Of course, the traditional 'spit' routine always works.

Accessories

When cleaning a handbag, remove the contents and stuff it with newspapers or plastic.

For leather or suede gloves, stuff the fingers with paper towels or empty toilet rolls. Place the gloves on top of a fizzy drinks bottle to dry.

Brush your jewellery with baking soda or toothpaste.

Use only the mildest soap when cleaning pearls.

Get your eyeglasses to stay put by dabbing clear nail varnish on top of the screws.

Organization

Take your earrings and fasten them through the holes of a button. This will keep them from getting separated.

Gather up all your brooches and pin them to a cork notice board. They will be in sight and available. No more rummaging in drawers for those jewels.

Use old stuffed cushions to create pin art. If you are a brooch collector, use a cushion for each colour theme, and you will have created a colourful display. After all, isn't jewellery art?

Use a hanger to display all your necklaces. This will eliminate the unnecessary tangling and knotting created by throwing long chains into jewellery boxes.

Miscellaneous

Use shampoo and conditioner you've never liked to wash your hair and make-up brushes. Shampoo and soak everything! Rinse with conditioner. They will be in soft, silky shape and will make your cosmetics and hair flow beautifully!

If any of your cosmetics start to smell different, then throw them away immediately. If you're on a budget, always look for oil-free cosmetics. They last a lot longer.

Eye make-up has the shortest shelf life. Because eyes are so easily irritated, eye make-up contains fewer preservatives. Keeping any eyeliner or mascara more than six months is putting you at risk of eye infections.

It's not necessarily a good deal to purchase larger containers. Bacteria build up if a product is not used right away.

Facts about Fragrances

Perfumes don't last forever. Once you open a bottle, use it until it's empty. Limit your perfume's exposure to the air. Fragrance is very much like wine; once it's open, it starts to disintegrate. Women who line their boudoirs with bottles of various fragrances will unfortunately find that eventually the quality will be jeopardized and some of them will sour. Once a perfume or cologne starts to smell like alcohol or vinegar, it's time to toss it.

Foods affect natural body odours and the fragrance of perfumes. That's why one scent will smell one way on a vegetarian, and another on a meat-eater. Fragrances will

147

smell differently on people who eat garlicky foods as opposed to those who eat more bland foods. Fragrance is also different at certain times of a woman's menstrual cycle. Other factors affecting your perfume's fragrance are vitamins, cigarettes and certain drugs.

Every night, plan to bathe in your favourite fragrance, and mend your mind from the day's stresses. Your bathroom is one room in your home that is made for sensory pleasures. Add a little mood music, and you've created your own aromatherapy experience. Don't forget the candles.

Chapter Fourteen

INTIMATE BEAUTY

Home Sweet Spa

Every woman deserves an area in her home that is entirely hers. If you do not have that space, begin to create one. It will be your own laboratory, where you can establish a home 'spa'. This area will be the one place you will use to store your own ideas and creations and try some of the tips that I will share with you in this chapter.

Make Your Own Toothpaste

In my work, I have come into contact with some inventive beauties and some real space cadets. Would you believe that there are some models using bathroom cleansers in an effort to whiten their teeth? These young beauties (who won't be lovely for long) are under the false impression that they can whiten their teeth with Comet and Ajax. Not only will this practice wear the enamel away, it is also dangerous!

There are secret recipes being passed around that WILL safely whiten your teeth, not cost you an arm and a leg, and not cause you to lose your enamel.

Burnt Toast

It may sound strange, but burnt toast is effective in whitening teeth. Pound a couple of slices into a powder and add a few drops of peppermint oil. The charcoal in the toast is the key ingredient.

Hydrogen Peroxide

Mix 1 teaspoon of hydrogen peroxide and 1 teaspoon of bicarbonate of soda. Brush your teeth with this mixture once a week. Be very careful not to swallow! This formula will reduce tarter and remove coffee and tea stains.

Salt

Mix 3 tablespoons of bicarbonate of soda with 2 tablespoons of salt for a safe and natural cleanser for teeth.

Do-It-Yourself Mouthwashes

Tea Wash

Boil a strong cup of mint (peppermint, spearmint, etc.) tea. Cool and rinse.

Honey/Clove Rinse

Mix 60ml (2fl oz) of honey with 1 teaspoon of ground cloves. This mouthwash can be thinned down if desired.

Agony of the Feet

What is it about feet? Some people love theirs, and there are some who will never show them, ever. Most of us just feel that our feet are not our best feature. We try to ignore them and rarely discuss them. Pedicurists report that clients come in with a list of apologies relating to their feet. How interesting that we feel that way about a potentially lovely part of our body. Properly cared for, the foot can become a major beauty asset. The foot is without a doubt the most neglected part of the anatomy. Historically considered an erogenous zone, feet are overdue for a rethink.

Wear the Proper Shoe Size

When purchasing a heel higher than 2.5cm (1in), go up half a size. Some natural swelling occurs that necessitates advancing at least half a size in order to accommodate the toe area. This is one time when smaller is not more attractive. A tight shoe bulges the foot out, not to mention what it does for the wearer's expression. A larger shoe actually gives the foot a longer, more graceful line.

Take Good Care

Use an antiperspirant on your feet. The foot contains more sweat glands than the underarm area. Don't waste that precious money on expensive foot powders and other foot remedies. Not only is this cosmetically important, but it is crucial in keeping bacteria at bay.

Change Shoes

Never wear the same pair of shoes two days in a row. Give them at least 24 hours to air out.

Soak Your Feet

At least once a week, steep 4 tea bags (purchase an inexpensive brand because it will contain a larger amount of tannic acid) in 460ml (16fl oz) of boiling water for at least 5 minutes. Add the same amount of cool water. Soak for up to 30 minutes. Note: Don't use herbal tea, because it's the tannic acid that will cause proteins in the skin to bond. This thickens the skin and blocks many of its sweat pores.

The Healthy Breast

Wear a Bra

The chest muscles don't provide enough support to go bra-less, no matter how small your breasts.

Keep your weight constant. Yo-yo dieting can cause the breasts to sag.

When trying on a bra, lean way over to make sure breasts fit snugly and comfortably in cups.

Eat Low-Fat Foods

It has not been completely discounted that eating high-fat foods could lead to breast cancer.

Exercise in the Proper Bra

If your breasts feel tender after a workout, you're probably not wearing a sports bra.

A sports bra should be made of material that prevents sweat from gathering underneath and between the breasts.

Make sure that the straps don't slip while running or jumping.

Perspiration

Perspiring can collect in the cleavage and especially under the bust. Keep the area dry by dusting the breasts with talcum powder before dressing.

Bulges

Should you find yourself 'pouring out' of your bra, choose a style with more support at the sides and underneath.

Bathing

The beauty benefits of bathing are many. Use bath time as a restorative, a spa and an occasion for dealing with intimate hygiene.

Temperature

Keep water warm, rather than hot. A too-hot bath will leave you feeling dehydrated and strips the skin of moisture.

Additives

Tea

Tie a tea bag under the tap so that the water will run through the bag. Use your favourite herbal teas, which will scent the water and you. The aroma will relax and invigorate you.

Alka-Seltzer

Toss a tablet into your bathtub and your bath will fill up with tiny bubbles, skin softeners and other good things.

Baby Oil

Soften water and your skin to silken elegance with a splash of baby oil.

Intimate Information

Hair Removal

Getting rid of hair is so much fun, isn't it? Here are some pointers that I hope will make the job a bit less tedious.

1. Don't shave right after getting out of bed. Skin tends to be puffy in the morning, and stubble is not as visible. Try to wait half an hour if you can.

2. Make sure hair is well-moistened. Use shaving cream, soap or other softener.

3. Start at ankles, go to bikini line and then to underarms. This gives coarser hair a chance to soften.

4. Avoid getting waxed just before or during your period. You are more sensitive to pain at this time.

5. Pluck hair in the bath-tub. It's easier to pluck when skin's warm and soft.

6. Shave opposite the direction of hair growth. It prevents hairs from curling under the skin and becoming ingrown.

7. Numb areas with witch hazel or ice to lessen pain.

The Bikini Area

The bikini line can be difficult to shave because the hair grows in so many different directions. Always prepare the skin with soap and water. Don't stop shaving the bikini area just because the colder months have set in, and you've stopped wearing a bathing suit. Discontinuing to shave this area will cause it to become overly sensitive. So when the warmer months return, you'll have to 'break in' that area again. OUCH!

Some women choose to shave or trim their pubic hair for hygienic purposes as well as appearance. Use caution when doing so. Use small scissors for safety.

Underarms

Hair also grows in different directions in the underarm area. Teach yourself to shave up and down AND sideways. Always prep this area thoroughly.

Deodorants

There are more deodorants on the market than ever. The truth about deodorants is that there's a lot of hype in the marketing. Sweat is sweat, whether it's on a man or woman. Models don't want to lose big jobs by ruining a designer dress with perspiration. You won't find any fancy, delicate flowery deodorants in a model's bag. Go get the strongest (yes, the ones made for a man) antiperspirant that you can find, and forget about the fancy, overpriced, weak stuff.

Tips for the Home

1. Stop paying for a cleaning woman. Blast that stereo, clean and exercise at the same time.

2. Choose underwear that matches your skin tone. Don't try to match your clothing.

3. Keep an aloe vera plant in your house. Break it open and use it to heal a sunburn. Apply it to your face as a refresher.

4. Grow parsley for fresh breath.

Loofah Your Legs

Try to give your legs a light scrub with a loofah before you shave them. This will get rid of all the excess dead skin cells that may otherwise clog up your razor. If you use a double-edged razor, then switch to a single-edged one.

5. Keep cucumbers for emergency eye compresses.

6. Stock up on bicarbonate of soda. Use it to soothe your skin in the bath. Brush your teeth with it. Clean your jewellery.

7. Rely on lemons to remove stains on teeth, soften hard skin on elbows and knees and rinse your hair.

Bloat

If you have a tendency towards excess bloating, don't chew gum, sip through a straw or drink from a bottle. These cause you to swallow air, which goes to your stomach.

Baring Skin

Make sure to wash after shampooing and conditioning your hair. Hair products leave a residue of oil on your shoulders and back. Always wear sunscreen on exposed chest and back areas.

Cellulite

The methods of getting rid of cellulite are controversial to say the least. The 'cottage cheese' that seems to gather on the back of the thighs and other spots is best eliminated by working it off in an aerobic programme. Spot exercises fail miserably. Running, walking, dancing, swimming and skating rev up the body's metabolism for burning fat throughout the body.

Work off cellulite in your bath-tub. Lie on your stomach, bend one knee, raise and lower heel to the ceiling. Try not to drown doing this exercise.

Some cellulite marks that are so unsightly can be diminished with massage. Break open a vitamin E capsule (1,000 units) with a safety pin, and rub into those troublesome areas.

Sex as a Health Tool

If you are a victim of irregular menstrual cycles, check your sex life. Researchers have found that women who have sex every week are more likely to have regular menstrual cycles of 28 or 29 days.

Women who have sex regularly find that their skin tone is better. This is due to the level of oestrogen being raised. It may in fact be the reason that people who are in love look so radiant. Increased levels of hormones are also said to cause hair to grow and shine. Sex is also a great stress reliever.

Sleep for Beauty

There can be no doubt about it. When we don't get enough sleep, we don't look well. Most of us need at least eight hours of uninterrupted sleep. Tossing and turning or awakening several times a night is detrimental not only to your looks but to your whole psyche. Unfortunately, it's not always so easy to fall asleep and stay asleep. But there are ways to put the odds in your favour.

Eat Early

There are very important reasons to eat dinner early, if possible before 8pm. Late-night eating makes for difficulty in sleeping. You will end up wide awake, while your body is trying to digest your last meal. If you've eaten certain kinds of food, you'll experience painful heartburn. Plus, as every successful dieter knows, those late meals are not good for weight reduction.

Scent Your Pillow

Add a few drops of eucalyptus oil (available at health food shops) to promote breathing. Stuffy nasal passages, whether due to a cold, flu or allergies, can cause you to awaken during the night. Scientists have discovered that when you have a cold, you awaken up to a hundred times, although you may not be aware of it.

Drink Tea

Several teas on the market today have been found to be helpful in inducing sleep. Although chamomile tea promotes sleep, it's also a diuretic, defeating its purpose.

Set Your Clock

Try to go to sleep and wake up at the same time every day, including weekends. Your body will try to adjust to a regular schedule. Sleeping in on weekends will disrupt your body's inner clock.

Sleeping on Your Back

Here's an age-old beauty secret which you won't pay a penny for but which could save you dozens of wrinkles over

159

the years. Wrinkles form on the side you sleep on. If you can't train yourself to remain on your back, invest in a satin pillowcase. Your face is going to slide around all night on this pillowcase, discouraging the wrinkling effect.

Keep It Cool

In an offbeat way, a slightly cool room is in fact, a beauty treatment. A room that is too hot can cause you to perspire. This increases oil production, which clogs the skin's pores. Equally important is to sleep on (and in) bed linen that 'breathes'.

Wash Off Your Makeup

PLEASE!! Remove every bit of face and eye make-up before getting into bed. Failing to do so can cause bacteria buildup and acne.

Get Plenty of Exercise

Although going through a rigorous workout routine just before bedtime can keep you awake, regular exercise may help you to sleep longer and more soundly. If you should find yourself 'wired', do some easy stretching to relax and soothe your muscles and promote a good night's sleep.

Take a Bath

A warm bath will relax the body into a 'ready for sleep' mode. Use bathing as a prelude to a night of beautiful dreams.

Get Gorgeous

Use the heaviest moisturizer you can find to make up for the loss of water during the night.

Fight free radicals during the night by puncturing a vitamin C capsule and adding it to your night cream.

Elevate your head with a firm pillow to eliminate puffiness.

Chapter Fifteen
SUPPLEMENTS

Supplements for Weight Loss

Garcinia Cambogia

Garcinia cambogia is a yellow fruit from Southeast Asia. Used in cooking, the garcinia extract is added to make meals more filling. Said to aid digestion, it contains hydroxyl citric acid, which is similar to the citric acid in citrus fruits.

Research conducted in the 1970s at Brandeis University, in the United States and later by Hoffman-LaRoche (the pharmaceutical company) showed that rats fed hydroxyl citrate shed 25 percent of their body fat in twenty-two days. The rats lost body fat partly because hydroxyl citric acid inhibits an enzyme that converts surplus carbohydrate calories into fat.

Available in pill form at health food shops, garcinia cambogia has taken the natural weight loss industry by storm. It controls the appetite in a natural, safe way, and has no side effects.

How to Take It

This is a supplement that is most effective taken thirty to sixty minutes before meals. Take it with a glass of water or with a piece of fruit. Taking it with a bowl of soup also seems to help.

Chromium Picolinate

Scientists have discovered that people who lack chromium in their bodies carry extra weight. The supplement chromium picolinate and chromium polynicotate have been around for a few years. It is an essential dietary nutrient which plays an important role in processing fat and carbohydrates. Many users report that it cuts sweet cravings, too. You could use this supplement if your diet lacks in chromium-rich foods. These foods include mushrooms, apples, broccoli and cheese. The recommended daily allowance is anywhere from 50 to 200 micrograms. Supplements are usually sold in 200 micrograms or mixed with other products in varying amounts. This product is readily available in drugstores, health food shops and in some chemists.

L-Carnitine

This supplement is reported to accelerate the benefits of chromium. Leading fitness buffs and die-hard weight watchers take the two together. It is sold as a separate unit and in combination with other supplements. L-Carnitine is an amino acid, that may be in short supply in many diets. The recommended dosage for this supplement is from 250 to 500 mg daily.

Supplements for a More Beautiful Life

Our attitudes have really changed toward supplements. I don't know of a beauty today who does not take her daily supply of vitamins and minerals in capsule form. For looks, vitality and general well-being, we models would have to consume too many calories if we were to rely on food during the day. That's why supplements are now playing such an important role in the regimens of the world's most beautiful women. However, it must be stressed that it is possible for most people to get all the vitamins and minerals they need by eating a well-balanced diet and most doctors would recommend this in preference to a reliance on supplements.

Here are the supplements most often mentioned as part of their daily diets. There is nothing you can apply external-ly that can compete with internal treatment of the body.

Vitamin A

Take this supplement to regulate skin hydration, aid eye-sight and repair skin and nails.

Vinegar

For thousands of years healers have used vinegar. Take two teaspoons of vinegar mixed with a glass of water at each meal. The vinegar will help your body to burn fat, rather than store it. Use any vinegar that appeals to you. Apple cider vinegar is a delicious flavour to try. Vinegar is a natural storehouse of vitamins and minerals. Give it a try.

Vitamin B

This important vitamin keeps skin smooth, promotes hair and nail growth and improves circulation.

Vitamin C

Available in several forms, it is quickly becoming the darling of the cosmetics industry. Vitamin C prolongs the life of vitamin E, and protects immune cells in the skin to fight off cancer and other sun-related diseases. It also has been proven to fade age spots and other pigment irregularities. Of course, vitamin C also fends off colds.

Vitamin E

Known as the skin vitamin, it has properties to heal scar tissue and neutralize damaging free radicals.

Ginkgo Biloba

Good circulation is vital to a healthy brain to supply it with the food and oxygen it needs. The ginkgo tree, derived from the oldest living tree, has many benefits. It increases alertness, improves memory and lowers cholesterol levels. But more importantly (to our looks) there's evidence that ginkgo may be the most potent anti-ager ever! The only problem I have come across is that there's no agreed-upon standard for the right amount to take. About 40 mg seems to be the recommended dosage from most sources I have consulted.

Beta Carotene

This vitamin A precursor protects cell membranes and skin cells from free radical attack. In everyday language, beta carotene makes the skin stay moist, supple and youthful.

Pycnogenol

A compound from the French maritime pine, this is a most powerful antioxidant which acts in a similar way to vitamin E, but with fifty times the strength. It boasts twenty times the strength of vitamin C. Use it to protect cell membranes from sun damage.

Grape Seeds

Antioxidants in grape seeds protect the thin walls of blood vessels from losing their strength. Beauties use it to prevent and correct the appearance of spider veins.

Echinacea

Rich in polysaccharides, echinacea helps to activate the immune cells. It naturally inhibits inflammation and is widely used in Europe. Take it only when you feel an illness coming on. It has no cumulative effects.

Licorice Root

Long used in Germany, this helps with vitamin absorption and the prevention of ulcers.

Seaweed

What you used to avoid at the beach has many health benefits. It's sold both in dried form and in tablets. You can reconstitute it and add it to your salads and soups as many models do. If seaweed doesn't exactly tempt your taste buds, go for the tablets. The most popular tablet is Kelp. Take it for its rehydrating benefits. Seaweed can also boost a sluggish thyroid.

Melatonin

This supplement is the ultimate sleeping pill, eliminates jet lag and improves mood. It is also reported to enhance the immune system, treat a variety of diseases and even prolong life. The biggest claims that have been reported (but which are as yet unproven), is that it can reverse the ageing process, fight cancers and even prevent pregnancy. However, while melatonin is readily available in the U.S. it is unfortunately still illegal in Britain. (Also see Chapter Fourteen).

Evening Primrose Oil

This very popular oil benefits the skin and hair and is said to aid in hair restoration.

Garlic

Take the deodorized version in table form to lower high blood pressure.

Lavender Oil

Use it in drop form in the bath to alleviate stress and ease headache pain.

Ginger

It prevents motion sickness and relieves nausea. Ginger is also reported to prevent and heal ulcers.

Grapefruit Seed Extract

Made from the seeds and pulp of grapefruits, grapefruit seed extract is receiving praise from both holistic and mainstream medical researchers. Its properties boost the immune system and are proclaimed to be an alternative to antibiotics. It is reported to fight bacteria, viruses and parasites, which is why it is most often used for flus, colds, sore throats and even yeast infections.

Bee Pollen

The buzz on bee pollen is that it gives you an extra energy lift. Be sure to take small doses of it in the beginning. Some users have found that they are allergic to it. It's used as an alternative to coffee by holistic groups.

Ginseng

This popular supplement has many health and longevity benefits. It improves energy levels and enhances mental alertness. It has immune strengthening benefits and can lower cholesterol levels. Ginseng is reported to decrease the chance of heart disease, and to increase good (HDL) cholesterol levels.

Dong Quai

Also known as dang gui and tang kuei, this is one of the most versatile herbs available today. From the name, it is obvious that its origins are in Chinese medicine. It has been used to treat menstrual problems (cramps, PMS) and menopausal symptoms. It is also useful in treating respiratory problems and even gas.

Selenium

Take this vitamin to enhance the effects of vitamin E. Selenium has a close metabolic interrelationship with vitamin E and aids in body growth.

Royal Jelly

Here is one of the most enduringly popular food supplements. Swathed in the mysteries of ancient China and the East, where it was first discovered, royal jelly in its raw state, is a unique, high protein food. It's produced by bees and fed to their offspring. Used as a food supplement, it is available in both capsule and liquid forms. Loyal followers prefer the liquid because it can be more easily absorbed into the system. Also use it to boost your energy levels.

Cat's Claw

Known as the Peruvian wonder herb, cat's claw is the newest herb to come out of the ancient rainforest of the Amazon. A natural antioxidant, it also offers the major benefit of being anti-oedemic (takes down swelling). Use it for swollen ankles, bloating and PMS.

Wheat Grass Juice

Here's yet another purported natural energy enhancer. It is also used in homeopathic healing of some diseases.

Spirulina

Used by weight-conscious beauties worldwide, spirulina is believed to dampen the appetite. It's widely available in health food shops, in many different brands, and is inexpensive and completely natural.

Silica

Many people swear by silica for radiant skin, luxuriant hair and rapid, strong nail growth. It also provides collagen to the body.

Coenzyme Q-10

Produced in the body naturally, it is being hailed as a powerful weapon against heart disease. Research also suggests that it may prolong youth and enhance the power of the brain. Mice given coenzyme Q-10 remained extremely active into old age and tended to live longer. The results did not come in until the mice grew old, which makes Q-10 more of an insurance policy than an overnight miracle.

Valerian Root

For those who can't take melatonin, valerian root is a useful alternative – as a mild tranquillizer and sleep aid.

Cranberry

Taken as a powdered concentrate, cranberry prevents recurrence of urinary tract infections.

The Best Time to Take Supplements

Although the specific hour is not really important, what is necessary is that you take your supplements at the same time each day. Make them part of your routine. Some supplements are better absorbed with food.

Chapter Sixteen
BEAUTY EMERGENCIES

What Beauty Crisis?

How do you handle a beauty emergency? You do it quickly and quietly. There's not one of you out there who has not had to deal with a crisis at one time. You stayed too long at that party, and it shows. The alarm didn't go off, and there's no time to get it all together. Well, it happens to movie stars, models and a lot of other celebrities we admire. There's nothing more traumatic to a model than being told you've been hired for the cover of the year and then coming down with the virus of the season. Tricks used to handle these emergencies are given in this chapter. Use them when you want to look your best but are feeling your worst.

Out, Damned Spot!

As models begin their careers at a young age, they quickly become experts in blemish disguise. There are ways to get rid of these 'party poopers'.

Eye Redness Reliever

This isn't just for eyes — it works on spots, too. Take any brand that 'takes the redness out' of the eye, and dab a bit onto a cotton swab. Hold it on the pimple for about a minute. These products take the redness away from the pimple, rendering it colourless and invisible. I would suggest that you also apply a little extra foundation or concealer in the general area of the pimple.

Toothpaste

Take just a little of your everyday toothpaste (not gel), and gently dab on the pimple, blending it well.

Calamine Lotion

Use it at night to take away the rashlike appearance of blemishes on face, neck, chest and back.

Ice Cube

Apply it directly on the pimple, and hold for several seconds. Follow up with a dab of 1 per cent hydrocortisone cream, available over the counter from chemists.

Covering Up a Cold Sore

There are medications for cold sores and fever blisters. If you don't have any on hand, take an aspirin and apply it, slightly dampened, to the sore. Hold it there for at least three minutes.

Keep the sore and its surrounding area clean and dry to fight bacteria.

Eat a bland diet, avoiding chocolate, nuts or gelatin-based products. These foods may irritate the sore and cause further infection.

173

Fresh Breath Fast

If you should find yourself without breath mints at the dinner table, don't panic! If there's parsley sitting on your plate, pick it up, and chew on it. Parsley has chlorophyll, similar to what you'll find in Clorets.

If you're drinking water, ask the waiter to bring it with lemon. Squeeze it into the water and drink up. The lemon will refresh your breath.

Chew some basil, ginger or mint leaves.

Eat a ginger biscuit.

Grab an apple! As you chew, you'll clean away any leftover particles of food caught between teeth.

Ask the waiter to bring you some bicarbonate of soda. Run to the ladies' room, and rub it over your teeth and tongue.

Tea Tree Oil

Massage a touch of tea tree oil around the area of a pimple to anaesthetize and encourage healing. Use a non-liquid concealer to match your foundation. Dab a little on the blemish, wait a couple of seconds, then blend lightly with a fingertip. Dust with loose powder.

Puffy Eyes

Spoon

Run a spoon under cold water, and place it over each eye. If you find your whole face swollen, open the freezer door. Stick your face in, and count to 100. Makeup artists have been known to do it to models who come in to a shoot looking a bit groggy.

Ice

Lie down and place plastic ice cubes or frozen teething rings on your eyes for about two minutes. Tap the area around the lids lightly with your fingertips.

Tea Bags

Run a couple of tea bags under hot water first, then cold water. Hold them over your eyes for at least five minutes.

Instant Colour

Cleanse your face. Then take two facecloths, one soaked in hot water, and one in cold water. Hold the hot cloth to your face for fifteen seconds, then the cold one for another fifteen seconds. Alternate the hot/cold treatment at least three more times. Your capillaries will expand, improving blood flow, tone and colour.

Using both hands, apply your moisturizer to your face, sweeping upwards. Gently pinch skin from the cheekbones to the jaw line. Tap on the face lightly with fingertips. Do this in an up-and-down movement from the neck, all the way to the edges of the forehead. Finish by quickly stroking the face with the pads of the fingers. Do it from the chin area right to the hairline.

Fill a basin with cold water, about twenty ice cubes and three tablespoons of witch hazel. Splash your face about ten times with this mixture.

Put two ice cubes into a plastic bag. Run it over your face several times until you begin to see some colour in your face.

Quick Fixes

Problem: A Headache Won't Go Away; Aspirin Is Not Available

Apply ice to your forehead and hold for about three minutes. If this doesn't work, try rubbing your scalp and temples with gentle but firm strokes.

Problem: You Have a Bad Case of 'Hat' Hair

If you can plan ahead when wearing a hat, don't apply too many styling products. After removing your hat, spray your hair with a little water. Then, tousle and shake until all the ridges disappear. Backcomb your hair gently from ends to roots.

If this still doesn't break a 'hat head', then add a bit of gel, and slick your hair back.

Problem: Your Hair Has 'Frozen'

This actually happens to many women during the cold months of winter, especially sports enthusiasts. First, don't touch your hair until it thaws. Your hair could actually break off! Then gently 'shake' your head until your hairstyle returns to normal.

Problem: Static Hair

If you ever find your hair catching onto your coat or the walls or standing on end when you attempt to brush it, always use a leave-in conditioner. If it's too late, slick on a bit of anti-frizz liquid.

Problem: Your Feet Are Aching after a Long Day

Add a few drops of eucalyptus or almond oil to your legs and feet. Massage it in, moving your thumbs in small circular motions.

Roll feet around on a bunch of small apples or marbles to ease away knots that come from wearing high heels.

Problem: You've Gone Too Heavy on Your Powder or Foundation

Squirt a little water on your face and lightly sponge off with a tissue.

Problem: You've Got No Time to Wash Your Hair

Dust it with powder or cornflour, and brush through.

If your hair is on the shorter, wavier side, take the front section of your hair, dampen it and divide it into four sections. Wrap each section around your finger and secure it with a clip. Dry hair on a low setting, and you'll achieve a fresh set of curls.

Tip your hair upside down, spray a gel on the under-growth and blow-dry. This will give new life and movement to your hair.

Still at the office? Take a soft-drink can and wrap your hair around it. Hold it in place with an elastic band. You probably won't have hair spray at your desk, so grab a little perfume (everyone should have a small container in her handbag) and spray.

Always carry a big black headband for worst-case scenarios. It looks chic, yet controls and smooths even the most unruly hair.

Problem: Those Roots Have Popped Up Out of Nowhere, and There's No Time to Colour!

Run for a box of chalk, and find a colour that most closely matches your hair. Don't think of using crayon. You'll never get it out!

If you have dark hair, use a matching mascara on the roots.

You can buy 'hair mascara' at cosmetic counters. This looks like ordinary mascara, only bigger, and comes in about ten shades.

Problem: Tired Eyes

Use navy mascara instead of the traditional black or brown. Most of us don't keep navy mascara on hand, so just rub any mascara into that old blue shadow. You should have thrown out that blue eye shadow by now, but it might be lurking somewhere in the back of your cosmetic drawer.

Soft colours like taupe and pink are better for tired eyes than strong dark tones.

Blue eyeliner applied along the rim of the bottom lid will make the whites of the eyes appear brighter.

Problem: You've Applied Your Eye Liner with Too Heavy a Hand

Soften the look by applying eye shadow in a co-ordinating colour over the liner. Blend together with a cotton bud.

If you use liner above AND below the eye, don't allow the two lines to meet. It will make the eye look too small.

Problem: Your Skin Is Red

If it's just your nose that's red, a little extra concealer in a darker tone will relieve it. Shade down the sides with a darker foundation to take away redness.

Problem: Big Under–Eye Circles

Mix a bit of blue eye shadow with moisturizer. Follow with foundation. Apply a concealer at least half a shade lighter than your skin tone. Use it after applying your foundation.

Is your entire face red? A bad sunburn perhaps? Smooth on a lotion containing at least 70 per cent aloe vera.

Apply a cold pack to your face.

To further neutralize redness, apply a yellow-based foundation, followed by a bronzing powder in lieu of blush and translucent powder.

Rub a strawberry over the redness.

Problem: You've Sprayed on Too Much Perfume

Dilute heavy fragrance by taking a warm, soapy facecloth to pulse points. Note: always apply scent to skin and not to clothing.

Problem: Nail Varnish Has Turned Nails Yellow

Apply white vinegar to the nail.

Problem: You've Lost a Button, or the Button Is Loose or Hanging

Should you find yourself with this problem at a restaurant or party, whisper to your host/waiter that you need him to retrieve a storage bag tie from the kitchen. Taking the tie, strip away all the plastic until there's just metal. Thread the button with the metal strip.

Use a binder clasp to replace a brass button.

Problem: You've Lost Your Cufflinks

Create a new pair with binder clasps from your office/

school. Everyone will want to know where you purchased those expensive brass cufflinks.

Use a pair of earrings for an elegant look.

Problem: There's No Time for a Manicure

If your varnish is just chipped, dip a cotton swab into some varnish remover. Pat it over the chipped area to smooth out. Touch up the area with matching varnish. Dry quickly by running the nail under very cold water.

Problem: Your Nail Varnish Has Become Dull

Coat your varnished nails with a drop of olive oil. Rub it into your cuticles as well.

Problem: You Don't Have Time for a Face Lift

Beat one egg white until frothy. Apply mixture to face and neck, and allow to dry. Rinse gently if you find that you've applied too much.

Lift your face with surgical tape, sold in most beauty supply stores. Stick it to the skin with spirit gum. If you only knew how many movie stars are doing this!

Problem: You're Wearing a Strapless Dress and You Need to Remove Strap Marks

Cover up lines with a tinted moisturizer or a foundation that is one shade darker than your skin tone. Use a sponge, and build up the colour gradually or evenly.

181

Problem: You're in a Hurry and Can't Start from Scratch

Don't take off any make-up if you're rushed, just intensify what's already there. Concentrate on retouching. Dot on concealer sparingly. Use a cotton bud to smooth out eye shadow creases. Add a touch of white or ivory to the brow bone (this wakes eyes right up). Comb eyelashes out (use a lash comb or toothbrush) and apply more mascara. Brush eyebrows and line them with a soft pencil.

Add bronzing powder to contour areas (jaw, cheek, sides of nose). Apply lip liner over existing lipstick. Powder over. Line lids again with a darker colour.

Problem: Those Eyebrows Are Just Too Dark

Go over the eyebrow with a concealer or light shadow.

Problem: You're Out of Concealer

Apply an extra coating of foundation. Use an ivory eye shadow.

Problem: You've Got Sweaty Palms

Apply a liquid or gel antiperspirant on your palms. Let it dry. A spray will work better than a roll-on. A powdery spray is best and takes only seconds to dry.

If you're in an office, just spray on a little perfume. The alcohol will absorb the perspiration in a pinch.

A small amount of talc will also work.

Problem: Static Cling

Slide a metal hanger over your tights, under

your skirt or blouse, or even over your hair.

The metal will neutralize the electric charge.

Problem: You Need to Wash and Dry Your Tights in a Hurry

Wash them in shampoo, and whirl them in a salad spinner to get rid of all excess water. Dry them with a 1200-watt hair dryer.

Problem: Your Trousers Are Too Tight to Tuck In

Fake a tucked-in look by tying a piece of string around the sweater or top, and pulling it over what will become a makeshift waistband.

Problem: Your Shirt Keeps Popping Out

Tuck your shirt into your tights.

Problem: Stains

White chalks will cover stains on white and light-coloured fabrics. Coloured chalk is good for all others.

For an unyielding stain, cover it with a brooch.

If there's time, sew on an appliqué motif, or use Velcro sequin decorations.

Problem: Too-Tight Waist

Secure a rubber band around the top button, pull it through the buttonhole, and loop what's remaining back on the button. You will need to camouflage this little trick by wearing a belt or long top. But, hey! you'll be comfortable.

Problem: Skirts That Won't Lie Down!

Make a small incision in the underside of the hem, and drop in a few small coins. The weight will help the skirt stay down and lie flat.

Problem: A Blouse or Jacket Gaps Open

Use double-sided tape to hold each gap together.

Problem: Shoes Are Too Big, and Slide Around

Line the shoe with a kitchen paper or pieces of tissue folded in thirds.

Problem: You Need to Shorten a Necklace

Shorten the necklace to the desired length, loop a small safety pin through the lines, and fasten. Tuck the dangling ends into the back of the shirt.

Problem: A Skirt Is Too Long

Roll over the waistband until the desired length is achieved. Keep it from rolling back down by belting it.

Problem: Bloodshot Eyes

Use blue eye make-up to take away the redness. Always stay clear of brown tones, because brown carries a strong red pigment.

Problem: Pierced Earrings Are Too Heavy

Take the eraser off a pencil and push it through the stem. It will hold the earring steady and upright on the ear.

Earring holes should be high enough to avoid accidental ripping of ear lobes.

Problem: Chapped Lips

Wet down lips with petroleum jelly. Remove flakiness with a toothbrush.

Problem: Your Iron Scorched Your Fabric

Hand wash the item in a basin of water together with 240ml (8fl oz) of hydrogen peroxide and a mild detergent.

Problem: You've Lost the Cleaning Instructions for That Expensive Dress

A reputable dry cleaner should be able to tell you about the care of the fabric. They will 'test' dry clean the fabric on an inconspicuous scrap.

Check with the shop where you bought it, and see if they can track down the garment's properties.

Problem: You've Left Your Makeup Pencils in High Heat and They've Become Mushy

Put them in a plastic bag and place in the freezer for an hour.

Problem: Shoe Polish Has Dried Up

Place the container in a bowl filled with hot water for a few minutes. Make sure that the tin is closed tightly before immersing.

Problem: A Big Ugly Wart Has Developed Overnight!

Puncture a vitamin A capsule, mix with a drop of lemon juice and apply it to the wart directly.

Problem: The Pool Has Turned Your Hair Green!

Dissolve ten aspirin in a cup of warm water and pour over hair. Leave on for five minutes.

Rinse in cool water.

Problem: Acne Rashes

Mix one packet of dry yeast with enough chamomile tea to make a paste. Spread it over the area. Let the mixture dry on your skin, and rinse.

Problem: Broken Spectacles

If a screw has fallen out of your eyeglasses or sunglasses, insert a wooden toothpick through the hinge as a temporary replacement. Break off the toothpick so that it will not show.

Problem: You Lose a Zipper Pull

Tugging on a zipper, the washing cycle, etc., can destroy a zipper pull. Hook a safety pin through it.

A dangling earring makes an attractive zipper pull.

Problem: Too Much Self–Tanner

Since self-tanning lotions can be tricky to apply, you could end up looking streaky. Use a body scrub for as long as it takes to fade away.

Use a light bronzing powder to disguise the zebra look.

Problem: A Bad Sunburn

Take an aspirin to help reduce the inflammation. Bathe in a tub of vinegar and warm water (use about 460ml [16fl oz] of any vinegar). Moisturize the skin with yoghurt or skimmed milk.

Problem: There's Not a Nail File to Be Found

Use the strip of a matchbox to file away snags.

Problem: Sore Eyes

In this high-tech world, sore eyes can be a real problem. Soak a pad in full-fat milk, and place on closed eyes for ten minutes. Rinse with cold water. The fat in full-fat milk has anti-inflammatory agents.

Problem: You've Lost Your Eyelash Curler

Use the back of a spoon. Some women prefer this method as a less tricky way to curl.

Problem: Knotted Jewellery

Lay the chain on a piece of greaseproof paper. Place a drop of olive oil directly on the knot. Use two needles to untangle the knots.

Problem: There's No One to Help You Fasten Your Bracelet

Tape one end of your bracelet to your wrist. It will stay in place so that you can attach the other end.

Problem: You've Used the Wrong Colour Dye in Your Hair

Tone down a too-bright colour by massaging a few drops of olive oil into dry hair, then covering hair with a shower cap for thirty minutes. Shampoo with a clarifying shampoo or even a mild washing-up liquid.

Chapter Seventeen
QUESTIONS

Miscellaneous Questions

Wherever I go, I seem to be asked the same questions. The following is a compilation of the most frequently asked questions and their answers.

How Do I Grow Out My Fringe?

Have your stylist add a few more long layers around the face. This will help fringes blend in subtly as they grow. The ends should be angled. Be patient, because it can take up to a year for fringes to grow to chin length.

How Do I Refresh My Makeup?
If I Add More Powder, It Looks too Cakey and Streaky.

Don't add more makeup until you've sprayed your face with some mineral water or toner. Then separate a tissue, and gently blot with both pieces. Your face will no longer have that 'stale' look, and you can add a bit more concealer, blusher, etc., on a fresher-looking face.

I'm Not Sure How Much of
My Lips to Colour. I Hate That 'Overdrawn' Look.

Form your lips into an 'O' shape. Your lipstick should go right to the edges with no gaps.

What's a Good Way to Line Eyes?

Look down into a mirror, and pull the lid taut. Draw a line as close to the lashes as possible. Start at the top centre of the lid, and go back and forth in short strokes. Be sure to go all the way to the outer lid with a final stroke pointing up, rather than down.

How Do I Make My Large Pores Look Smaller?

After cleansing your face, apply a toner to tighten pores. Use an oil-free foundation, making certain to blend evenly. Pat on powder, using a large puff for the most even coverage.

Is It Acceptable to Wear Leather All Year Round?

It's impossible to wear leather in tropical temperatures. Leather holds heat, and will cause great discomfort. What you wear with leather will dictate its wearability into warmer weather. Short-sleeved cottons and silks are good choices.

How Can I Prevent My Nails from Chipping?

Apply a strengthening top coat the day after a new manicure. Continue to apply another coat every other day until your next manicure.

How Can I Make My Office Wardrobe Appear Polished and Professional without Looking Boring?

You need to add some lighter colours and softer cuts and fabrics to your wardrobe. A dress with a matching jacket is a softer alternative to the traditional suit. Also consider wearing a tailored dress. With the right accessories, it can look both professional and feminine.

Why Do I Always Break Out in Red Bumps after I Shave My Legs?

Try exfoliating your legs with a coarse facecloth or loofah before shaving.

What Is a Safe Way to Straighten Naturally Curly Hair?

Use a jumbo-sized curling iron, and keep its temperature at about 38°C (100°F). If your iron doesn't have a temperature dial, try not to keep it so hot that you can't touch it.

How Can I Make My Fragrance Last Longer?

Start by 'layering' your scent. Begin with a scented shower or bath laced with your signature fragrance. Next, apply perfumed body lotion to slightly damp skin. Finish off by applying perfume to your pulse points.

How Do I Know That I'm Buying a Good Moisturizer?

Head to your local chemist and start reading labels. Check to see the ingredients that these and their pricier counterparts have in common; these are increasingly being listed on cosmetic labels in Britain, as they are in the States. You'll be pleasantly surprised to learn that many are very similar in their listing.

How Can I Make My Eyes Look Pretty without Shadow?

Apply foundation one or two shades darker than your regular foundation. Finish with black mascara.

How Do I Grow Out a Perm?

Have it cut into long layers, trimming the most damaged parts.

How Can I Make My Eye Shadows Look Less Fake?

Use 'cream' or 'cream to powder' finishes. They don't require an exact application and blend in less conspicuously.

When I Line My Eyebrows, They Look Very Harsh.

To achieve a more natural look avoid using any eyebrow liner. Switch to an eye shadow in your brow's colour or slightly darker.

I Like 'Smoky' Eyes, but I Can't Get It to Look Good.

The look of black-rimmed eyes belongs on the runways. Use your eye shadow as a liner by wetting it. It stays on longer than other eyeliners and will look softer.

How Can I Make My Nails Grow?

Eating a well-balanced meal, high in calcium, is all you need to think about. Take at least the recommended dosage of calcium daily.

Will Cutting My Hair Make It Grow Faster?

No; unfortunately, just cutting your hair will not make it grow any faster. Getting regular trims WILL keep the ends strong and thick. This will make it appear that your hair is longer and stronger.

Why Does a Perfume Smell Great on My Sister and Terrible on Me?

Your body chemistry reacts to perfume in a unique way. There are other factors to consider as well, such as diet, medication and even the weather. Always test a fragrance, and then walk around for about 20 minutes before making a purchase.

How Do I Get Rid of Flaky Skin?

Be sure to exfoliate your skin at least three times a week. This will remove all the dead surface cells that accumulate, and will provide a smooth surface on which to apply your makeup.

What Goes on First, Concealer or Foundation?

This is a personal choice, but it does look more natural when concealer is mixed with a little bit of foundation.

Is It Okay to Wear Open-Toed Shoes in Winter?

It's perfectly all right to wear open-toed shoes as long as you're wearing sheer, sandal-foot tights, and a special-occasion dress.

Why Do I Get Tiny Bumps on My Arms?

People with dry skin or eczema tend to get these bumps, which are caused by hair follicles that become clogged with oil and dead skin. When you notice them, apply an acid-based body moisturizer. This will help clear out pores.

Why Is My Hair Colour Changing?

It could be your water. If you've moved home recently, you may have gone from soft to hard water. Hard water can cause blonde hair to take on a greenish cast, while causing brown hair to run red.

What's the Best Way to Add Volume to Flat Hair?

Let hair air dry, then roll it up in large Velcro rollers. Spray hair with a volumizer and blow dry directly over rollers.

How Do I Prevent Lipstick from Getting on My Teeth?

After applying lipstick, seal it in with a bit of blusher in a co-ordinating colour.

I Like the Look of Leggings, but I Don't Like My Legs. What Can I Do?

Wear stretch trousers that contains a combination of wool, cotton, rayon and Lycra. They will hold you in without emphasizing bulges.

What Can I Do with Leftover Shampoos?

Use them as bath gels. They'll do the job and clean your tub too. You can also use unwanted shampoo to wash delicate fabrics.

I Like Nude Tights, but My Legs Don't Look Attractive in Them.

The secret of wearing nude tights is to match the colour of your tights to your arm colour. Most women choose their tights based on their leg colour. This looks too pale and causes the legs to look lighter than the rest of the body.

How Do I Know Where to Pluck My Eyebrows?

Hold a pencil vertically so that it rests beside your nose. The spot where the pencil meets the brow is where the eyebrow should begin. Pluck any stray hairs outside of that area.

I'm a Large-Sized Woman. How Do I Select Trousers?

Stay away from elastic waistbands. Although comfortable, they are not flattering. Instead, look for a single-pleat or flat-panelled style in a fluid fabric.

What Can I Do to Keep My Lips from Drying Out?

Keep yourself hydrated by drinking lots of water. Also, slick a little bit of honey on your lips. Not only is honey rich in moisturizers, but it also provides a protective barrier.

Besides Drinking Coffee, Is There Anything I Can Do at Work to Avoid Mid-Afternoon Slump?

Revive tired muscles and stimulate blood flow by placing a plastic mineral water bottle on the floor. Take off your shoe, and gently roll your foot over it from your heel to your toes. Repeat with the other foot.

Can I Use a Topcoat on Nails as a Base Coat?

These products are not as similar as they may seem. Base coats are thicker than top coats. This is one case where it's necessary to stick to the recommended use.

How Can I Prevent White Flaky Stains on My Clothing Caused by My Deodorant?

Use solid stick deodorants; they are usually less messy than roll-ons.

I Have a Linen Suit That I Love. How Can I Keep It from Creasing?

Try hanging it in the bathroom, and let the steam smooth out most of the creases.

What Can I Do to Keep My Rings from Turning My Finger Green?

Always apply hand cream before wearing your rings. This forms a barrier between the skin and the metal.

Chapter Eighteen
FABULOUS FIGURES

YOU Can Be Fit and Fabulous!

Is there a magic elixir that will help you drop the weight that keeps you from getting your body into the shape you've always dreamed of or used to have? I have tons (sorry)! To start with, women and men who make their fortunes from their looks are real people. In between photo shoots, movies, appearances, etc., they like to party, gain a few pounds, and enjoy their lives. That includes eating well. But they do take care of those inevitable kilos that they will gain BEFORE the kilos have a chance to accumulate. There are amazing secrets among trainers, agents and the stars themselves who are the very cutting edge of the industry. Taking this information and incorporating it into your lifestyle will definitely make the difference for you. Just be sure to make these changes gradually, and you will be successful in finally taking charge of your body, your health and your life.

Dieting Is Dead!

The idea is to change the way you look at food, so that you'll be healthier, and stay thinner. Be intelligent about food, and be certain that whatever you eat you will end up wearing.

What Do You Want to Weigh?

The weight ranges for men and women have recently changed. This is the latest chart to date. Realize that it's not just the kilos that count, it's how you carry them. If you are constantly trying to reach a goal that's 2–4kg (5–10lb) below what you currently weigh, then maybe you're not meant to be that weight. But first, look at your lifestyle. Is that Friday-night pizza party more important than the fit of your jeans? It's a tough question that only YOU can answer.

Healthy Weight Ranges for Men & Women

152cm	(5' 0")	44–58kg	(6st 13–9st 2)
155cm	(5' 1")	46–60kg	(7st 3–9st 6)
158cm	(5' 2")	47–62kg	(7st 6–9st 11)
160cm	(5' 3")	49–64kg	(7st 9–10st 1)
163cm	(5' 4")	50–66kg	(7st 13–10st 6)
165cm	(5' 5")	52–68kg	(8st 2–10st 10)
168cm	(5' 6")	54–70kg	(8st 6–11st 1)
170cm	(5' 7")	55–73kg	(8st 9–11st 6)
173cm	(5' 8")	57–75kg	(8st 13–11st 10)
175cm	(5' 9")	59–77kg	(9st 3–11st 13)
178cm	(5' 10")	60–79kg	(9st 6–12st 6)
180cm	(5' 11")	62–81kg	(9st 10–12st 11)
183cm	(6' 0")	64–84kg	(10st–13st 2)

Women should try to get their weight to the bottom range for their height.

Heights are indicated for measurement without shoes.

Weigh yourself in the morning, before breakfast and without any clothing.

Top Secrets

Iced Water

Ask any woman with a body to die for what her secret is, and most likely she will tell you that she drinks lots of water. That is so true, but it's only half the story. It's the ice that you add to your water that really makes the difference. Drinking iced water forces your system to rev up your metabolism, to keep the body's temperature from dropping. For example, if you drink eight 350ml (12fl oz) glasses of iced water a day, your body will burn an additional 200 calories.

Drink water consistently throughout the day. By the time you are really feeling thirsty, you are on your way to becoming dehydrated.

Often what we think of as hunger is thirst. If you find it difficult to down water in large quantities, flavour it up with a bit of lemon or lime. Water can provide a feeling of fullness and help the kidneys and liver do their job.

Don't be fooled into thinking that drinking lots of water will bloat you. Water retention is more likely to be caused by not drinking enough.

Seeds

To maximize your intake of nutrients, add a lot of seed-containing fruits and vegetables such as apples, pears and bananas, as well as the seeds themselves (like sesame or sunflower seeds). Seeds are a great source of fibre, allowing foods to go through your body quickly.

Spicy Foods

Scientists have discovered that chilli, peppers, salsa, mustard and ginger can actually raise your metabolic rate. The result is that you can burn calories much faster; up to 45 per cent faster than on a bland diet. How? These foods create a thermogenic burn, meaning they help the body to produce 'heat', thus burning off calories.

Herbs That Help Shed Kilos

There are herbs you can add to your diet as supplements, teas and foods that will help your weight loss programme go smoothly.

Alfalfa
Aids digestion and acts as a diuretic.

Bladderwrack
Improves thyroid function and is a bulk laxative.

Burdock
Improves fat metabolism and acts as a diuretic.

201

Cardamom

Improves circulation and digestion. A thermogenic herb.

Cayenne

Improves circulation and digestion. Has thermogenic effects.

Cinnamon

Creates a thermogenic burn.

Dandelion Root

Aids fat metabolism by affecting the liver.

Fennel

A diuretic that reduces hunger and improves energy.

Flax Seed

A bulk laxative that helps curb hunger.

Garcinia Cambogia

Aids fat metabolism and reduces hunger.

Green Tea

Aids fat metabolism and increases energy.

Hawthorn

Reduces blood fat and improves circulation.

Parsley

A diuretic and nutritional aid.

Senna

An all-natural laxative.

Foods for the Skin

A diet for a fabulous you includes foods for great skin!

Blueberries

Promote healthy collagen for fewer wrinkles. Less constriction of veins and faster healing.

Carrots

Contain high levels of beta carotene for protection against sun damage.

Salmon

Rich in essential fatty acids to keep skin moisturized.

Eggs

High in the amino acid *cystein*, necessary for the growth and maintenance of the body's tissues.

Sweet Potatoes

Rich in vitamin A to protect the skin from environmental damage.

Mushrooms

Rich in selenium, an antioxidant that may help lower skin cancer risks.

Yoghurt

Contains vitamin B complex which is essential for smooth, blemish-free skin.

Reasons to Eat Breakfast

1. You'll have a better day at work. Women who eat breakfast work faster and more accurately than those who don't. Breakfast-eaters are also more creative in the morning.

2. It keeps you in shape. Breakfast-eaters are slimmer than those who skip breakfast. They don't reach for doughnuts or croissants at the first coffee break.

3. You'll have lots of health benefits. Cereal with skimmed milk and fruit boosts your vitamin intake for under 200 calories.

How to Get the Most from Your Meals

Lay a Beautiful Table

Choose one or two places in the home at which to eat. Make each meal a special occasion. Eat only at these places, and never eat while standing.

Don't Play that Funky Music

Don't ever eat a meal to toe-tapping tunes. Researchers have found that diners who listen to classical music take three bites a minute as compared to five bites a minute with rock music. They also enjoy their meal more thoroughly and feel more satisfied.

No TV

To be truly enjoyed, eating requires full attention. Turn off the TV and put away that reading.

Chew Away Tension

Relax your facial muscles, and satisfy your chewing urges by chewing slowly. It takes fifteen minutes for your brain to communicate to your stomach that it's full.

Small Is Smart

Choosing to eat meals on smaller plates can fool the eye, which relates to tricking the brain into thinking that it's devoured a plateful.

Add Flavour, Not Calories

Discover flavoured vinegars to add flavour without the calories. Use a tablespoon of vinegar to thin down and extend your favourite dressings.

Add salsa to just about any food. It perks up the taste buds with little or no fat. Dip vegetables in it, spoon it over scrambled eggs or baked potatoes, and add it to salads.

Keep olive oil in a spray bottle and add it to salads, vegetables and even popcorn.

Say It with Soya

Soya is packed with powerful antioxidants which interfere with free radical damage. This is the basis for how fast we age. Soya is another reason to turn to a more vegetarian-based diet. Unlike animal proteins, soya beans don't spew scads of damaging free radicals through your body to age your cells. Soya also prevents heart disease and diabetes. Japanese, who eat the most soyabean in the world (thirty times more than Americans, for example) live longer than anyone. Soya is also reported to cut breast cancer rates and to lower blood cholesterol.

Satisfy Your Sweet Tooth

When you desire something sweet, don't grab that chocolate bar. Try a natural sweet such as grapes, raspberries or strawberries.

When fruit just won't do, go for a jelly bean. At only six calories each, these fat-free sweets are one of the modelling world's favourite snacks

How to Deal with Cravings

Brush Your Teeth

That awful taste you have in your mouth when restricting calorie intake can lead to eating. Instead, brush your teeth and tongue with a flavoured toothpaste.

Focus on Fragrance

Enjoy foods for their fragrance, as well as their appearance and taste. Studies have proven that we obtain a great deal of satisfaction from a food's smell.

Do Something Else

Have a bath or go to a movie. Go for a walk or phone a friend. Do anything until that hungry feeling goes away. Don't worry, eventually those cravings will subside.

Drink Water

Add a lot of lemons to take away that awful empty feeling that cravings bring.

Eat Bread

Sometime a single slice of bread can calm nerves and end that craving as no other food can.

Rest

It may be that you just need to relax for a few minutes. Don't try to restore your energy level with food.

Get Your Protein

A small protein-rich snack can eliminate that craving by keeping blood sugar and energy levels balanced.

Watch Out for Allergies

It may not be the food you're craving that's the culprit. Get checked for allergies to wheat and dairy.

Are You Sure It's Hunger?

There are physical signs that will let you know if you're just experiencing a craving or if you're really hungry.

1. Headache, a lightheaded feeling or irritability
2. A need for any carbohydrate
3. Increased salivation
4. Stomach noises

Your Refrigerator

Did you know that the refrigerator is opened on an average of twenty-two times a day? Since it's such an integral part of our dining plans, here's how to make sure this appliance is not abused.

Stick a Mirror on It

Buy a mirror that attaches to the front of the refrigerator (or stick one on with Blu-Tak). You'll find that if you have to face yourself each time you peek in, it just may wake you up to reality.

Tape Up an Inspirational Note

Make that note a trigger for your success. 'I can do it' or 'Just a month until swimsuit season'.

Hang Up a Picture of What You Want to Look Like

It could be a photo of you when you looked your best. It might be a picture of your favourite celebrity. Paste YOUR head onto a supermodel's body.

Keep the Fat in the Fridge

Take 500g (17½oz) of butter and keep it in a plastic bag. Make it the first thing you see when you open that refrigerator.

Portion All Your Foods

Pack all your food in bags. You'll see your daily allotment at a glance. Knowing that you're limited to those bags provides a focus.

More Tips

Red wine

Drinking a glass of red wine can speed up metabolism rates.

Lollipops

Sucking a lollipop can calm nerves and stop sugar cravings.

Sugarless Sweets

Sweets containing artificial sweeteners can't be broken down in the body efficiently and can cause severe bloating.

Stomachs Can Shrink

After a period of restricting calories, the stomach's capacity will actually decrease.

Tensing

No need to stay at home with an expensive exercise machine when you can tense your stomach muscles in and out wherever you are!

The Fat Test

If you want to know if a food is high in fat but the packaging isn't handy, rub the food with a paper napkin.

If it leaves a grease mark, it's probably got more fat than you want.

Be Prepared

When travelling, always carry something healthy to eat and drink. It will steer you away from vending machines and fast-food restaurants.

Cut Back on Calories Without Counting

Eat Treats

If you don't treat yourself now and then, you'll just crave it more. This will lead to an unfortunate binge.

Leave Out the Fat

Chances are that many of your favourite foods can remain in your diet if you cut back on cheese, butter, cream, etc.

Spread It Out

Salad dressings, spreads, etc., can be thinned out with vinegars, yoghurt and other low-fat extenders.

Check Your Portions

Weigh and measure your foods when it's convenient.

Stop Late Night-Eating

Your body can't digest those late-night snacks when it's at rest.

Don't Drink Your Calories

Learn to like low-calorie drinks for painless calorie cutting.

Eat Like a Grown-Up

Start experimenting with exotic foods that are low in calories. For instance, try some of the more unusual mushrooms now available in supermarkets, such as giroles and oyster mushrooms. Leave those old fat-filled cheeseburgers to the kids.

Don't Skip Meals

You'll end up eating twice as much, and your metabolism will be messed up with low bloodsugar levels.

Shop with the Right Attitude

Never go shopping for food when you're ravenous. You'll end up with all the wrong stuff in your trolley.

What's In Your Coffee?

Since there are so many speciality coffees around, be certain that you're really ordering a potentially delicious, refreshing low-calorie drink.

Regular or decaf	4 calories
Espresso	5 calories
Cappuccino	40 calories
Latte	60 calories
Café mocha	150 calories

Jump-start Diets

The clock is ticking, and there are just a few days to that special event. Or perhaps you hate the thought of a long, dreary diet. You need motivation with quick visible results.

You can make those two or three kilos disappear. Stars and models do it all the time. And you can too!

If you've put on a few pounds, it's very easy to take it off quickly with these 'jump-start' techniques. Plus, it just might be the motivation you need to get going towards a more significant weight-loss.

The Garlic and Papaya Diet

This is the one I use as a natural diuretic when I need to get someone into an outfit quickly and safely.

Take two garlic tablets and two papaya tablets before breakfast, lunch and dinner. Ask your pharmacist for the strongest strength available over-the-counter. Eat lightly for two days, staying away from salt, bread and fizzy drinks. Stay near a loo because this will draw fluids (safely) from your body.

The Cleansing Diet

Go on a diet of vegetables for two days. Start with toma-to juice and grapefruit juice for breakfast, and eat an array of greens for lunch and dinner.

The Watermelon Diet

For two days, eat several slices of watermelon with lots of water for breakfast and lunch. Eat a light, but nourishing, dinner. The film actress Ann Margaret reportedly used this diet for two weeks and lost 9kg (20lb). I wouldn't try this one for more than two or three days.

The Cabbage Diet

This diet has been passed around forever. It's been called the Model's Diet, the Stewardess's Diet, even the Dolly Parton Diet. I don't really know whose diet it is, but lots of people have had tremendous success with it.

Diet Soup Recipe

2 or 3 bouillon cubes
1 packet onion soup mix
3 onions
1 to 2 heads of cabbage
1–1.5kg (2–3lb) of tomatoes
1 carrot
1 sweet pepper
Seasonings to taste

Blanch tomatoes in boiling water for one minute. Plunge into cold water, remove skins and set aside. Dissolve soup mix and bouillon in 2 litres (3½ pints) of water. Chop then add cabbage, onion, carrot, pepper and spices. Add tomatoes. Bring to the boil and cook for 30 to 40 minutes. Makes enough soup for two days.

Eat all the Diet Soup you want for seven days along with the following:

1st day: fruits only
2nd day: vegetables only
3rd day: fruits and vegetables
4th day: bananas and skimmed milk
5th day: 170g (6oz) lean poultry or fish and plain rice
6th day: same as 5th day
7th day: vegetables and rice

Chapter Nineteen
RECIPES UNDER 200 CALORIES

Enjoy Your Favourite Foods!

The following recipes are real food! These are recipes that you would be proud to serve your family and friends. They are all easy to make, with products that are readily available. I encountered lots of difficulty in researching recipes for this chapter. Many recipes that were allegedly 'slimming' were anywhere from 500 to 600 calories per portion. Why bother? Other recipes had as many as twenty to twenty-five ingredients. If you're like me, you would not attempt to cook with that many steps. Our lives are just too busy, and we're too hungry to wait! What you'll love about this chapter is that each of the following recipes is a doddle to make and absolutely delicious! You can mix and match until you get the number of calories you'd like to consume for any particular day.

I've tried to include something for everyone's taste. The last thing you would find me doing is to tell you to eat cauliflower if you hate it. There are also some low-fat goodies for those of us who just can't end a meal without something sweet.

Enjoy!

APPETIZERS UNDER 200 CALORIES

Hot Spinach Artichoke Dip

95 calories per serving
Makes 24 servings

110g (4oz) grated Parmesan cheese
230ml (8fl oz) reduced-calorie mayonnaise
400g (14oz) artichoke hearts, drained and chopped
280g (10oz) frozen chopped spinach, thawed and drained
2 tablespoons chopped tomato
Garlic, salt and pepper to taste

Heat oven to 180°C (350°F; gas mark 4). Mix all ingredients, except tomato. Spoon into 23cm (9in) pie or quiche dish. Bake 30 to 35 minutes or until lightly browned. Serve topped with tomato.

Stuffed Mushrooms

41 calories per serving
Makes 4 servings

12 large mushrooms
2 tablespoons lemon juice, divided
1 small red onion, chopped
1 teaspoon fresh dill
2 tablespoons virtually fat-free plain yoghurt
1 teaspoon mustard (preferably Dijon)
Salt and pepper to taste

Finely chop mushroom stems, leaving caps whole. Over high heat combine 1 tablespoon lemon juice with 1 litre (1³⁄4 pints) water. Bring to the boil. Add mushroom caps and cook until tender. Transfer to a bowl filled with cold water. Drain and pat dry. Combine red onion, dill, yoghurt and mustard. Evenly divide filling among mushroom caps.

Creamy Leek Dip

65 calories per serving
Makes 10 servings

450g (16oz) low-fat cottage cheese
60ml (2fl oz) skimmed milk
1 packet leek soup mix
1 cup fresh parsley sprigs

In a food processor fitted with its metal blade, combine all ingredients except parsley sprigs until smooth. Add parsley and process until it is finely chopped. Place in a medium-sized bowl and refrigerate for at least 2 hours.

Salsa Dip

60 calories per serving

Makes 24 servings

450g (1lb) processed cheese spread

230g (8oz) salsa

Microwave cheese spread and salsa in a 2-litre (3 1/2-pint) microwave-safe bowl. Heat for 5 minutes on high. Stir after 3 minutes. Serve with baked tortilla chips, pepper wedges or baked potato skins.

Baked Onion Rings

51 calories per serving
Makes 4 servings

6 tablespoons seasoned dry bread crumbs
1/2 large sweet yellow onion
1 egg white

Preheat oven to 230°C (450°F; gas mark 8). Slice onion as thinly as possible. Separate into rings. Dip onion first in egg white, then bread crumbs. Place on a nonstick baking sheet. Bake 10 minutes.

Crab Meat Spread

28 calories per serving
Makes 12 servings

230g (8oz) crab meat
60g (2oz) celery, diced
1 small onion, diced
1/2 green pepper, diced
1 cup bean sprouts
170g (6oz) low-fat cottage cheese
Vinegar

Blend all ingredients using enough vinegar to moisten. Season to taste.

SOUPS UNDER 200 CALORIES

Gazpacho

52 calories per serving
Makes 6 servings

1 cucumber peeled, cut, and seeded
2 1/2 cups fresh tomatoes

1 large green pepper, chopped
1 large onion, chopped
1 teaspoon garlic flavouring
1 teaspoon dried chives
1 teaspoon paprika
Salt and pepper
1/2 teaspoon sugar
470ml (16fl oz) tomato juice
2 tablespoons lemon juice

Shred cucumber with grater. Combine tomatoes, pepper, onion and seasonings. Stir in remaining ingredients. Cover and chill at least 2 hours before serving.

Yellow Pepper & Orange Soup

35 calories per serving
Makes 4 servings

2 yellow sweet peppers, halved and seeded
1 large onion, chopped
Grated rind and juice of 1 orange
350ml (12fl oz) chicken stock
4 chopped olives
Salt and pepper to taste

Preheat grill. Place peppers skin side up on baking sheet. Grill until skins are blackened. Cover and leave to cool. Place onion and orange juice in pan. Bring to the boil, then cover and simmer 10 minutes. Peel peppers. Blend with onion, half orange rind and chicken stock. Season to taste, then heat gently. Serve sprinkled with olives and remaining rind.

Vichyssoise

149 calories per serving
Makes 6 servings

3 medium leeks
3 potatoes, peeled, and diced
700ml (1¼ pints) chicken stock
460ml (16fl oz) evaporated skimmed milk
Freshly ground pepper

Cut and discard roots and tough leaves from leeks. Cut
leeks in half lengthwise, and rinse under cold water. Then
cut leeks crosswise, into 5mm (¼in) thick slices. Spray a
saucepan with oil. Heat the pan over medium heat. Add
leeks, cooking and stirring for 5 minutes. Reduce heat
and simmer 30 minutes. Transfer leek mixture to food
processor. Blend until smooth. Stir in milk and pepper.
Soup may be chilled before serving.

Vegetable Soup

75 calories per serving
Makes 8 servings

460ml (16fl oz) tomato juice
460ml (16fl oz) water
400ml (14fl oz) chicken stock
450g (16oz) peeled tomatoes
230g (½lb) French beans cut into 2.5cm (1in) pieces
340g (¾lb) carrots, sliced
3 celery stalks, sliced
1 onion, sliced
1 courgette, sliced
1 yellow courgette, sliced

Combine tomato juice, water, stock and tomatoes. Bring to boil. Add French beans, carrots, celery, onion and courgette. Bring to boil, and simmer 30 minutes. Season to taste.

Cappelletti Soup

105 calories per serving

Makes 4 servings

700ml (1¹/₄ pints) beef stock

100g (3¹/₂oz) fresh cheese or meat cappelletti

150g (5oz) frozen peas

2 tablespoons sun-dried tomatoes

1 teaspoon dried basil

In a medium-sized saucepan, combine all ingredients. Cover and bring to boil. Reduce heat and simmer 5 minutes or until cappelletti are tender.

Mixed Bean Soup

95 calories a serving
Makes 4 servings

1 teaspoon olive oil
1 red onion, chopped
1 crushed garlic clove
170ml (6fl oz) tomato purée
1 teaspoon dried thyme
150g (5oz) frozen or fresh French beans
420g (15oz) tin cannellini beans
Salt and pepper to taste

Heat the olive oil and sauté onion and garlic until tender but not brown. Add the tomato purée and thyme, and bring to boil. Add the French beans, cover and simmer for about 6 minutes or until tender. Add cannellini beans and season.

SALADS

Greek Salad

90 calories per serving
Makes 2 servings

2 handfuls cos lettuce, torn into pieces
2 tablespoons feta cheese
1 tomato
1 cucumber
1/2 stalk celery, sliced
2 black olives
2 tablespoons vinegar
1 tablespoon olive oil

Toss all ingredients together, and serve.

German Potato Salad

180 calories per serving
Makes 4 servings

680g (1 1/2lb) small red potatoes
3 shallots or leeks, minced
2 tablespoons each of parsley, chives and thyme
2 tablespoons balsamic or wine vinegar
2 tablespoons beef stock
2 tablespoons olive oil
2 minced garlic cloves

Boil potatoes in saucepan until tender. Remove from heat, drain and cut in halves. In medium-sized bowl, toss with shallots or leeks and herbs. Set aside. In a small saucepan, combine vinegar, stock, olive oil and garlic. Warm over low heat and pour over potatoes. Fold in carefully before serving.

Red Coleslaw

40 calories per serving
Makes 4 servings

1/2 small red cabbage, shredded
1 red onion, thinly sliced
4 radishes, thinly sliced
1 red apple, cored and grated
1 tablespoon low-fat plain yoghurt
1 teaspoon honey
Salt and pepper to taste

Place cabbage, onion, radishes and apple in salad bowl. Toss. In a screw-top jar, shake the remaining ingredients until they are blended. Pour the dressing over the salad, toss and serve.

Couscous Salad

105 calories per serving
Makes 4 servings

170g (6oz) couscous
1 celery stalk, chopped
$1/2$ small cauliflower, cut into small florets
4 spring onions, chopped
3 tablespoons dried parsley
1 tablespoon lemon juice
$1/2$ teaspoon Tabasco
Salt & pepper to taste

Cook couscous according to instructions on packet. Leave to cool. Stir in remaining ingredients, season and toss. Spoon onto a large platter and serve.

Deli Salad

180 calories per serving
Makes 8 servings

200g (7oz) artichoke hearts, drained
170g (6oz) cubed mozzarella cheese
110g (4oz) fusilli pasta, cooked and drained
80g ($2^1/2$oz) pitted olives
115ml (4fl oz) low-fat vinaigrette or Italian dressing
1 large red onion, sliced
$1/2$ green pepper, chopped
30g (1oz) Parmesan cheese, grated

Mix all ingredients together. Refrigerate before serving.

224

Spinach Salad

80 calories per serving
Makes 4 servings

2 handfuls fresh spinach
170g (6oz) dried apricots, chopped
2 tablespoons sunflower seeds
1 tablespoon sesame seeds
2 tablespoons orange juice
1 tablespoon balsamic vinegar
2 tablespoons low-fat plain yoghurt
Salt and pepper to taste

Mix all ingrdients together. Refrigerate before serving.

Waldorf Salad

60 calories per serving
Makes 10 servings

680g (1 1/2lb) diced apples
280g (10oz) thinly sliced celery
90g (3oz) raisins
1.3 litres (2 1/4 pints) reduced calorie mayonnaise
60ml (2fl oz) half-fat crème fraîche

Combine apples, celery and raisins in a large bowl. Stir to mix well. In a small bowl, combine mayonnaise with crème fraîche. Stir. Add mayonnaise mixture to apple mixture, and toss together. Refrigerate for 2 hours before serving.

Chicken and Pasta Salad

165 calories per serving
Makes 8 servings

700ml (1¼ pints) chicken stock
450g (1lb) boneless chicken breasts
230g (8oz) of shell pasta
230ml (8fl oz) mayonnaise
1 teaspoon mustard
½ teaspoon celery salt
Freshly ground pepper
2 stalks of celery, thinly sliced
170g (6oz) petit pois, cooked, drained and cooled
170g (6oz) red grapes, washed, and cut in half

Bring stock to a simmer in medium-sized saucepan. Add chicken breasts and cook for 20 minutes. Remove breasts and chill. Cook pasta according to instructions, drain and rinse in cold water. Mix together mayonnaise, mustard, celery salt and pepper. Cut chicken into bite-sized pieces, and add to mixture. Add pasta, celery, peas and grapes. Toss together. Cover and refrigerate 1 hour.

Cucumber Salad with Dill

50 calories per serving
Makes 4 servings

2 cucumbers
3 tablespoons vinegar
1 tablespoon sugar
1 red onion, sliced and split into rings
Salt and pepper to taste
1 teaspoon dried dill weed (from health food shops)

Wash the cucumbers, and partially remove peel in length-wise strips. Use a fork to leave a little skin between each strip and slice crosswise. Combine vinegar, sugar, salt and pepper in a bowl until sugar is dissolved. Add cucumber, onion and dill. Toss well. Serve immediately.

VEGETABLE DISHES

Mange-tout Peas and Carrots

80 calories per serving
Makes 4 servings

1 onion, thinly sliced
4 teaspoons olive oil
2 carrots, cut into 5cm (2in) strips
230g (1/2lb) mange-tout peas, strings removed
2 teaspoons dried dill weed (from health food shops)
Salt and pepper to taste

Microwave onion and oil for 1 minute. Stir in carrots, cover with plastic and microwave for 2 minutes. Stir in mange-tout and dill. Microwave covered for 6 minutes. Let stand for 3 minutes. Season and serve.

Carrots and Grapes

45 calories per serving
Makes 4 servings

230g (8oz) sliced carrots
1 shallot, chopped
60ml (2fl oz) water
2 tablespoons red wine vinegar
1 tablespoon brown sugar
90g (3oz) halved seedless grapes

Cook carrots and shallot in water in nonstick frying pan about 10 minutes. Stir until carrots are tender. Push carrot mixture to side of pan. Stir in vinegar and sugar. Gently stir in grapes. Toss all together.

Potato Skins with Salsa

49 calories per serving
Makes 16 servings

Preheat oven to 230°C (450°F; gas mark 8).

4 baking potatoes
Salt and pepper to taste
1 small tomato, chopped
110g (4oz) black beans, drained and rinsed
2 tablespoons spring onions
1/2 teaspoon ground cumin
60g (2oz) grated reduced-fat cheddar cheese
230g (8oz) salsa
230g (8oz) plain virtually fat-free yoghurt

Prick potatoes and bake until tender (about an hour). Cool 15 minutes. Quarter potatoes lengthwise. Scoop out flesh, leaving the shells intact. Place skins on baking sheet sprayed with oil. Sprinkle with salt and pepper. Combine tomato, beans, spring onions and cumin. Sprinkle skins with cheese. Bake until cheese melts (about a minute). Top skins with salsa. Serve with yoghurt.

Vegetable Salad

55 calories per serving
Makes 8 servings

450g (1lb) broccoli, chopped
450g (1lb) cauliflower, chopped
110g (4oz) sliced celery
20 pitted, sliced black olives
430g (15oz) tinned mushrooms, drained
170ml (6fl oz) fat-free vinaigrette or Italian Salad dressing

Combine all ingredients in a large bowl. Stir to cover vegetables. Chill for at least 3 hours before serving.

Zucchini Frittata

65 calories per serving
Makes 4 servings

2 small courgettes
1 teaspoon water
2 spring onions, chopped
1 teaspoon basil
1 teaspoon dried marjoram
6 eggs
2 tablespoons Parmesan cheese

Cut each courgette lengthwise into quarters. Thinly slice each quarter. Place the water in a 25cm (10in) frying pan. Add courgettes and onions. Cook over low heat about 3 minutes. Discard cooking liquid. Stir in basil and marjoram. Beat eggs lightly with a fork, and carefully pour over courgettes and onions. Cook over low heat until mixture starts to set. Lift edges of uncooked mixture to flow underneath. Continue cooking until nearly set. Sprinkle with cheese. Grill 1 minute and serve.

Peas and Onions

105 calories per serving
Makes 8 servings

450g (1lb) small onions
2 tablespoons butter
570g (1¼lb) frozen peas, thawed
2 tablespoons chopped mint
1 tablespoon Parmesan cheese
Salt and pepper to taste

Peel onions, prick them through centre, and boil them in enough water to cover until tender. Drain. Melt butter in frying pan, and cook 3 minutes. Add onions and peas. Place in bowl, and toss with mint, cheese, salt and pepper.

Rosemary 'Fries'

75 calories per serving
Makes 4 servings

Preheat grill

3 large baking potatoes
2 teaspoons olive oil
1 teaspoon dried rosemary
Salt and pepper to taste

Cut potatoes lengthwise into 3 slices each. Cut each slice into 3 large chip shapes. Cook potatoes in microwave with a bit of water. Take out while still crisp (not mashing soft). Spread steamed potatoes on baking sheet sprayed with cooking oil. Sprinkle with dried rosemary. Grill until potatoes are golden brown. Turn and brown other side. Season and serve.

Glazed Carrots

70 calories per serving
Makes 4 servings

450g (1lb) carrots
230ml (8fl oz) water
4 teaspoons apple juice
1 tablespoon brown sugar
Knob of butter
1/2 teaspoon nutmeg

Cut carrots into 5cm (2in) pieces, then quarter length-wise. Microwave carrots in water for 5 minutes until just tender. Meanwhile, stir together apple juice, sugar and butter. Microwave for 30 seconds or until sugar and butter just melt. Drizzle carrots with juice mixture. Toss to coat. Serve sprinkled with nutmeg.

Rice Amandine

115 calories per serving
Makes 6 servings

1 large onion, chopped
280ml (10fl oz) chicken stock
1 tablespoon lemon juice
1/2 teaspoon garlic powder
285g (10oz) brown rice
230g (8oz) frozen green beans, thawed
2 tablespoons toasted flaked almonds
1/2 teaspoon dried dill weed

Cook rice following instructions on packet. Spray medium saucepan with cooking oil. Add onion and cook until tender. Add stock, lemon juice and garlic powder. Bring to boil. Stir in rice and return to boil. Reduce heat to low. Cover and simmer about 5 minutes. Remove from heat and stir in remaining ingredients. Fluff with fork and serve.

Swiss Asparagus au Gratin

170 calories per serving
Makes 4 servings

Heat oven to 200°C (400°F; gas mark 6).

120ml (4fl oz) water
680g (1¹/₂lb) asparagus spears, trimmed
60g (2oz) Swiss cheese, grated
30g (1oz) bread crumbs
30g (1oz) butter, melted
¹/₂ teaspoon dry mustard
¹/₄ teaspoon fresh ground pepper

Bring water to boil in 25cm (10in) frying pan. Add asparagus. Cook 2 minutes and drain. Place in 25 x 15cm (10 x 6in) roasting tin. Mix remaining ingredients Sprinkle over asparagus. Bake 10 minutes until cheese mixture is lightly browned.

MAIN DISHES UNDER 200 CALORIES

Grilled Flank Steak

170 calories per serving
Makes 4 servings

450g (1lb) lean flank steak
180ml (6fl oz) dry red wine
3 garlic cloves, cut into quarters
Bay leaf, cut in half
¹/₂ teaspoon onion salt
2 teaspoons Dijon mustard

Preheat grill. Marinate steak in a baking dish with wine, garlic and bay leaf for 1 hour. Drain steak. Place steak in a grill pan. Sprinkle with onion salt. Spread a thin layer of mustard over top. Grill to desired doneness.

Pineapple Steak Kebabs

185 calories per serving
Makes 4 servings

1 tablespoon soy sauce
2 tablespoons water
1 teaspoon garlic powder
1 tablespoon applesauce
450g (1lb) steak, cut into 5cm (2in) squares
Small red pepper, cut into 3cm (1in) squares
Unsweetened pineapple chunks
8 fresh mushrooms

Combine soy sauce, water, garlic powder and applesauce. Marinate steak 1 hour. Alternate steak, pepper, pineapple and mushrooms on skewers. Grill to desired doneness.

Pork Steaks with Peppercorn Glaze

175 calories per serving
Makes 4 servings

4 lean pork loin steaks
1 tablespoon green peppercorns, crushed
4 tablespoons balsamic vinegar
230ml (8fl oz) chicken stock
4 spring onions, sliced

Mix together peppercorns and vinegar. Sprinkle over pork. Let sit for 30 minutes. Reserving the peppercorn mixture, fry the pork in a nonstick pan. Add the peppercorn mixture, stock and spring onions. Boil rapidly, uncovered, for about 10 minutes.

Lemon Chicken

130 calories per serving
Makes 4 servings

Preheat oven to 180°C (350°F; gas mark 4)

4 boneless chicken breast halves
2 lemons
1 teaspoon dried tarragon
Fresh pepper to taste

Place chicken in foil-lined roasting tin. Fold sides of the foil up. Halve lemons and squeeze juice of 1/2 lemon over each chicken piece. Sprinkle each piece with 1/4 teaspoon tarragon and some pepper. Fold foil together, and seal to secure chicken. Bake for about 45 minutes.

Mediterranean Turkey Spirals

125 calories per serving
Makes 4 servings

4 thin turkey breast steaks
2 tablespoons pesto sauce
4 tablespoons basil leaves
115ml (4fl oz) chicken stock
240ml (8fl oz) tomato juice
Garlic salt and pepper

Pound turkey until thin. Spread with pesto sauce. Lay basil leaves over each steak, then roll in Swiss roll fashion. Secure with cocktail sticks. Combine stock and tomato juice. Bring to the boil over high heat. Add the turkey spirals, cover and simmer for 15 minutes. Season and remove cocktail sticks. Serve hot.

235

Turkey Meat Loaf

175 calories per serving
Makes 8 servings

Preheat oven to 180°C (350°F; gas mark 4).

680g (1¹/2lb) turkey breast
30g (1oz) seasoned bread crumbs
100g (3¹/2oz) uncooked rolled oats
115ml (4fl oz) semi-skimmed milk
2 tablespoons soy sauce
1 large onion, chopped
1 egg
Freshly ground pepper

Combine all ingredients. Place mixture in a loaf tin coated with cooking spray. Bake about 1 hour. Meat should not be pink.

Oysters Rockefeller

90 calories per serving
Makes 4 servings

Preheat grill.

2 teaspoons olive oil
1 tablespoon grated onion
2 tablespoons bread crumbs
Tarragon, pepper and Tabasco sauce to taste
280g (10oz) frozen chopped spinach, thawed and drained
230g (8oz) oysters, raw or tinned
2 tablespoons grated mozzarella cheese
1 tablespoon Parmesan cheese

Combine bread crumbs, oil, onion and seasonings. Toss mixture with spinach. Grill oysters for 5 to 7 minutes if raw. (Drain liquid if using tinned.) Top oysters with spinach mixture, and grill about 4 minutes. Sprinkle with cheeses and grill until just melted.

Devilled Prawns

140 calories per serving
Makes 1 serving

5 tiger prawns, uncooked, peeled and deveined
2 tablespoons white wine
1 tablespoon Dijon mustard
1 crushed garlic clove
2 tablespoons diced onion
Salt and pepper to taste
1 tomato, peeled
2 tablespoons chopped parsley

Spray frying pan with cooking oil. Add prawns and sauté about 2 minutes on each side. Add wine, mustard, garlic, onion and seasonings. Cover and cook about 8 minutes. Add tomato, breaking it up with a fork. Mix all together, cover again and cook 10 minutes. Add parsley and serve.

Baked Scallops

125 calories per serving

Makes 4 servings

Preheat oven to 230°C (450°F; gas mark 8).

1 tablespoon butter

60ml (2 fl oz) white wine

Juice of 1 lemon

450g (1lb) scallops

Combine, and heat all but the scallops in oven. Pour liquid over scallops. Marinate for 20 minutes at room temperature. Bake for about 15 minutes. Do not overcook.

Seafood Bisque

130 calories per serving
Makes 8 servings

340g (12oz) frozen sweetcorn, thawed
460ml (16fl oz) chicken stock
1 tablespoon butter
2 red or green peppers chopped
2 tablespoons chopped onion
Salt and pepper to taste
240ml (8fl oz) semi-skimmed milk

230g (¹/₂lb) prawns, cooked or raw, peeled and deveined
230g (¹/₂lb) scallops
3 tablespoons parsley

In food processor, combine 280g (10oz) sweetcorn with half the chicken stock. Purée until smooth. Melt butter over medium heat in saucepan. Add peppers, onions, salt and pepper to taste. Cook 5 minutes. Stir in sweetcorn mixture, milk and remaining stock. Cover and simmer 5 minutes. Add prawns, scallops, remaining sweetcorn and parsley. Cook about 5 minutes and serve.

Baked Aubergine, Tomatoes and Feta

95 calories per serving
Makes 4 servings

Preheat oven to 200°C (400°F; gas mark 6).

1 medium, thinly sliced aubergine
Garlic salt
2 large tomatoes, sliced
170g (6oz) crumbled feta cheese
4 tablespoons plain yoghurt
Olive oil
Paprika
Garlic salt

Sprinkle the aubergine slices with garlic salt, leave for 30 minutes, then wipe off. Spray baking dish with cooking oil. Arrange aubergine and tomatoes to overlap slightly. Sprinkle with feta cheese and spoon over yoghurt. Sprinkle with paprika and garlic salt. Bake for 30 minutes or until bubbling and golden.

Vegetarian Stuffed Peppers

145 calories per serving
Makes 6 servings

Preheat oven to 190°C (375°F; gas mark 5).

6 red or green peppers
300g (10^1/$_2$oz) cooked rice
60g (5^3/$_4$oz) cooked couscous
3 egg whites
Salt and pepper to taste
Parsley to taste
30g (1oz) seasoned bread crumbs
1 small onion, chopped
30g (1oz) chopped celery
230ml (8fl oz) passata

Cut peppers in half, and remove seeds. Microwave 2 minutes. Combine rice, couscous, egg whites and seasonings. Sprinkle in bread crumbs and set aside. Bring 240ml (8oz) water to boil. Add onion and celery and boil 15 more minutes. Add passata, mix and cook 20 minutes. Spray a baking dish with cooking oil. Fill peppers with stuffing. Cover with sauce. Bake for 40 minutes.

BREADS, PIZZA AND QUICHE UNDER 200 CALORIES

Lemon Pepper Popovers

105 calories per serving
Makes 6 servings

Preheat oven to 230°C (450°F; gas mark 8).

110g (4oz) flour
240ml (8fl oz) skimmed milk at room temperature
1 tablespoon olive oil

Salt and pepper to taste
2 teaspoons lemon zest
3 egg whites, slightly beaten

Mix together flour and milk. Add remaining ingredients, stirring until just mixed. Grease muffin cups with cooking spray. Fill each cup half full. Bake 15 minutes, then reduce heat to 180°C (350°F; gas mark 4) for 20 more minutes. Serve at once.

Blueberry Muffins

123 calories per serving
Makes 12 muffins

Preheat oven to 200°C (400°F; gas mark 6).

230g (8oz) plain flour
1 tablespoon baking powder
$1/2$ teaspoon salt
140g (5oz) blueberries
4 egg whites
350ml (12fl oz) virtually fat-free yoghurt
110g (4oz) sugar
1 teaspoon vanilla essence

Mix together flour, baking powder and salt. Add blueberries. Stir lightly to coat and set aside. Beat egg whites to peaks. Add yoghurt, sugar and vanilla. Add liquid mixture to dry ingredients and fold together gently. Bake for 20 minutes in nonstick 12-cup muffin tin.

Optional: Place 1 blueberry in the centre of each muffin. Sprinkle a little sugar over each muffin. Bake for 20 minutes.

241

Spiced Carrot Bread

125 calories per serving
Makes one loaf or 12 slices

Preheat oven to 180°C (350°F; gas mark 4).

2 eggs
4 tablespoons vegetable oil
3 tablespoons sugar
3 carrots, coarsely grated
140g (5oz) plain flour
1 teaspoon baking powder
2 teaspoons allspice
3 tablespoons skimmed milk

Line loaf tin with greaseproof paper. Mix together eggs, oil and sugar. Stir in carrots. Add flour, baking powder and allspice. Fold in milk. Pour into tin. Bake 40 to 45 minutes.

Spicy Onion Tart

175 calories per serving

Preheat oven to 190°C (375°F; gas mark 5).

1 tablespoon butter
4 large yellow onions
230ml (8fl oz) half-fat crème fraîche
3 eggs
Salt, black pepper and cayenne pepper to taste
1 frozen flan case
1 teaspoon dried parsley

Melt butter in large nonstick frying pan. Add onions. Cover and cook 15 minutes. Uncover and cook until browned. Remove from heat and let cool. Combine crème fraîche, eggs, peppers and salt. Add onions. Pour into flan case. Sprinkle with parsley. Bake 30 to 35 minutes. Cool slightly before cutting.

Grilled Crispbread

100 calories per serving
Makes 12 servings

Preheat grill.

230g (8oz) plain flour
1 teaspoon salt
4 tablespoons butter, melted
120ml (4oz) warm water
1 teaspoon paprika
Salt and pepper to taste

Combine flour and salt. Stir in 2 tablespoons butter. Stir in water 1 tablespoon at a time. Divide dough into 12 pieces and roll each piece into a circle. Spray baking tray with cooking oil. Grill circles for 2 minutes on each side, brushing with remaining butter. Sprinkle with salt, pepper and paprika. Grill one more minute.

DESSERTS UNDER 200 CALORIES

Lemon Bars

150 calories per serving
Makes 24 bars

Preheat oven to 180°C (350°F; gas mark 4).

230g (8oz) white vegetable fat
170g (6oz) brown sugar
170g (6oz) plain flour
1 teaspoon baking powder
1 teaspoon cinnamon
90g (3oz) quick-cooking oatmeal
230g (8oz) light cream cheese, softened
110g (4oz) granulated sugar
120ml (4fl oz) lemon juice
2 teaspoons grated lemon peel

Beat together vegetable fat and brown sugar. Add flour,
baking powder and cinnamon. Stir in oats. Reserve one-
fourth of oatmeal mixture. Press remaining oat mixture
onto bottom of greased 33 x 23cm (13 x 9in) pan. Beat
cream cheese with granulated sugar, juice and peel. Pour
over oat mixture. Sprinkle with remaining mixture. Bake
about 30 minutes.

Apple Crumble

135 calories per serving
Makes 8 servings

Preheat oven to 190°C (375°F; gas mark 5).

4 sliced apples
60g (2oz) brown sugar

30g (1oz) plain flour
30g (1oz) rolled oats
1 teaspoon cinnamon
2 tablespoons butter, softened

Spray a 20 x 20cm (8 x 8in) pan with cooking oil. Place apple slices in pan. Mix remaining ingredients together. Sprinkle over apples. Bake 30 minutes.

Baked Pizza

95 calories per serving

Makes 2 servings

1 large pitta bread

4 tablespoons pasta sauce

4 tablespoons low-fat cottage cheese

1/4 teaspoon dried oregano

1/2 teaspoon Parmesan cheese

Split bread in half horizontally.

Grill until toasted. Cover each half with sauce.

Follow with cottage cheese. Sprinkle with oregano and Parmesan cheese. Grill until cheese melts.

Apple Nut Biscuits

75 calories each
Makes 14 biscuits

Preheat oven to 200°C (400°F; gas mark 6).

140g (5oz) rolled oats
1 teaspoon allspice
4 tablespoons white vegetable fat
3 tablespoons brown sugar
1 apple, cored and chopped
3 tablespoons walnuts
1 egg white

Mix together oats, allspice and vegetable fat. Add sugar, apple, walnuts and egg white. Stir. Form 14 balls. Arrange on nonstick baking tray. Flatten slightly. Bake for 10 minutes.

Chocolate Truffles

60 calories per truffle

90g (3oz) chopped raisins
2 tablespoons chocolate-flavoured liqueur
40 digestive biscuits ground to a powder
405g (14oz) tin sweetened condensed skimmed milk
60g (2oz) unsweetened cocoa powder
1 teaspoon vanilla

Combine raisins and liqueur. Let stand until softened. Combine digestive biscuits, milk, half cocoa powder, vanilla and raisin mixture. Chill one hour. Place remaining cocoa powder in shallow bowl. Shape chocolate mixture into balls. Roll in cocoa powder. Freeze 15 minutes. Store in refrigerator.

Biscotti

65 calories per biscuit

Preheat oven to 180°C (350°F; gas mark 4).

340g (12oz) plain flour
1 teaspoon baking powder
140g (5oz) sugar
5 tablespoons white vegetable fat
3 eggs
1 tablespoon lemon juice
1 cup currants
110g (4oz) dried apricots

Combine flour and baking powder. Set aside. Cream together sugar and vegetable fat. Beat in eggs. Add lemon juice. Add dry ingredients. Add currants and apricots. Divide and shape dough into 2 loaves. Bake 30 minutes. Leave to cool and slice.

Cheesecake Cups

129 calories per serving
Makes 8 servings

Preheat oven to 190°C (375°F; gas mark 5).

950ml (33fl oz) low-fat yoghurt
1 teaspoon lemon juice
3 tablespoons granulated sugar
2 slices pumpernickel bread
2 tablespoons honey
1 cup mandarin orange sections

Strain yoghurt and refrigerate 4 hours. Stir in lemon juice and sugar. Refrigerate another 4 hours. Toast bread, crumble and add honey. Press into bottoms of eight muffin cups to make crust. Cover with yoghurt mixture. Add a couple of mandarin orange sections on top. Bake 15 minutes or until firm.

Fruit Skewers with Mango Purée

80 calories per serving
Makes 4 servings

1 ripe mango, peeled, pitted and chopped
1 tablespoon lime juice
1/2 cored pineapple
1 papaya, peeled and seeded
2 kiwi fruit, peeled and quartered

Place mango and lime juice in a food processor and blend. Cut pineapple and papaya into bite-sized chunks and thread on skewer with kiwi.

Note: To serve, spoon a little mango purée on four plates. Place cooked skewer on top.

Molasses Biscuits

50 calories per biscuit
Makes 40 biscuits

Preheat oven to 190°C (350°F; gas mark 4).

115ml (4fl oz) light molasses
75g (2 1/2oz) white vegetable oil
230g (8oz) plain flour
40g (1 1/2oz) brown sugar
1 tablespoon skimmed milk
1 teaspoon ginger
1/2 teaspoon baking powder

Heat molasses to boiling, and stir in fat until melted. Remove from heat, and stir in flour, sugar, milk, ginger and baking powder. Stir until mixture pulls away from pan. After dough cools, form into 3cm (1in) thick log. Refrigerate until firm. Slice into 5mm (1/4in) slices. Bake on nonstick baking tray for 10 minutes.

Chapter Twenty
THE INTERNET

Cyber Beauty

There is a wealth of valuable beauty, fashion and health information waiting for you on-line. You can even shop via computer. If you own a computer, all you need is a modem and a phone.

Magazines Online

Most UK magazines now have their own website. Not only will you be able to read this month's edition, but you can also search back to previous issues and articles.

Health-Related Sites

Do not substitute health sites for medical advice, but be sure to check them out.

Chapter Twenty-One
A FINAL WORD

It is my sincere hope that you will use this book to take charge, not only of your looks but of your life. No amount of make-up, clothing or cosmetic surgery can make you beautiful. The REAL secret of beauty is to live life with passion and compassion. Love as hard as you can and, yes, even allow yourself to feel the pain that will visit all of us.

There is no amount of make-up that will mask the life you've led. Let the spirit of your face show that you've lived your life with pride, grace and courage. Don't be afraid to try something new, to continually re-invent yourself during your days here on Earth. Certainly, don't allow your looks to rule your every waking moment. The key to true beauty is do the best you can and value yourself as much as you expect others to value you. Then go on. Do the very best that you can with all the other adventures of your life.

INDEX

About the Author

Diane Irons is a model, talk show host and internationally known fashion and image journalist who has worked with stars in the entertainment and fashion industries. She has appeared on national American radio and TV, including Maury Povich, Montel Williams, CNBC and Lifetime Television.